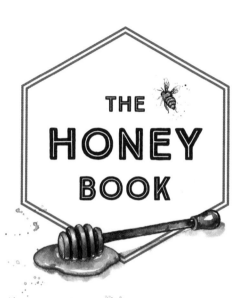

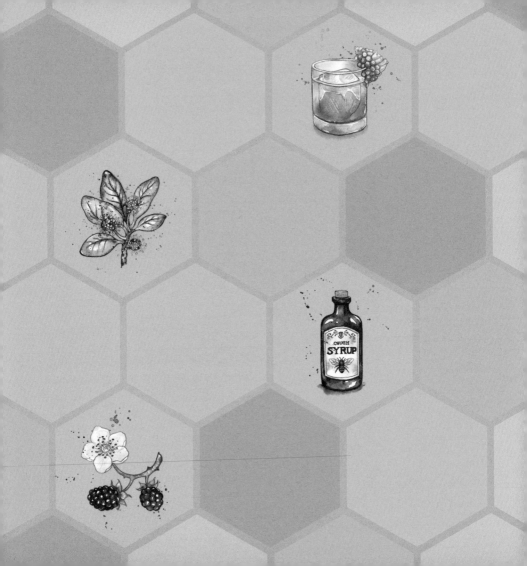

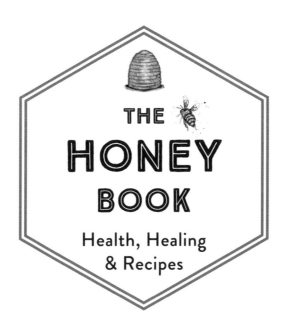

THE HONEY BOOK

Health, Healing & Recipes

ANDREA KIRK ASSAF

Illustrated by Amy Holliday

HarperCollins*Publishers*

**Dedicated to all queen bees, honey kings, and bee buddies –
and most especially to Honey King TJD**

HarperCollins*Publishers*
1 London Bridge Street
London SE1 9GF

www.harpercollins.co.uk

HarperCollins*Publishers*
1st Floor, Watermarque Building, Ringsend Road
Dublin 4, Ireland

First published by HarperCollins*Publishers* in 2021

1 3 5 7 9 10 8 6 4 2

Copyright © HarperCollins*Publishers* 2021

Andrea Kirk Assaf asserts her moral rights as the author of this work.

Text by Andrea Kirk Assaf
Cover and interior illustrations by Amy Holliday
Cover and interior design by Jacqui Caulton

A catalogue record for this book is available from the British Library

ISBN: 978-0-00-843011-5

Printed and bound in Latvia

All rights reserved. No part of this publication may be reproduced, stored in a retrieval system, or transmitted in any form or by any means (including electronic, mechanical, photocopying, recording, or otherwise) without prior written permission from the publisher.

Disclaimer:
The information in this book is not intended to be taken as a replacement for medical advice or the services of trained and qualified health professionals. Any person with a condition requiring medical attention should consult a qualified practitioner. While very rare, an allergic reaction to honey can occur in some individuals with pollen allergies. If this happens, consult a doctor immediately. It is not recommended to give honey to children under one year old.

MIX
Paper from
responsible sources
FSC™ C007454

This book is produced from independently certified FSC™ paper
to ensure responsible forest management.

For more information visit: www.harpercollins.co.uk/green

CONTENTS

CHAPTER ONE — 7
The surprising history and lore of honey

CHAPTER TWO — 29
The many sources and flavours of honey

CHAPTER THREE — 47
A honey buyer's guide – how to avoid fool's gold and find the real deal

CHAPTER FOUR — 65
Food and drink recipes with honey

CHAPTER FIVE — 107
Honey healthcare and beauty recipes

CHAPTER SIX — 125
Honey wisdom

Additional Resources — 135
Index — 142

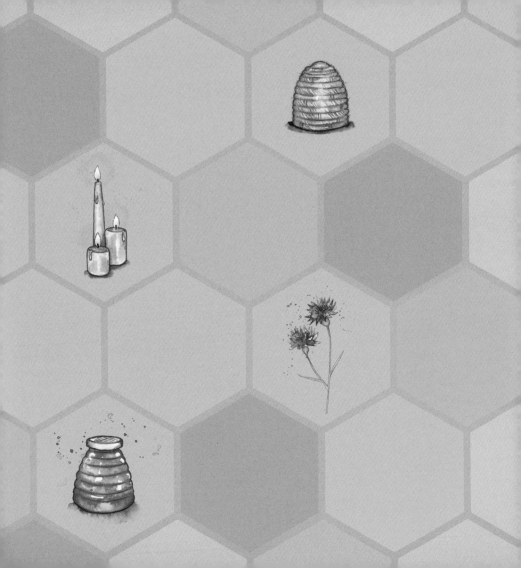

CHAPTER ONE

THE SURPRISING HISTORY AND LORE OF HONEY

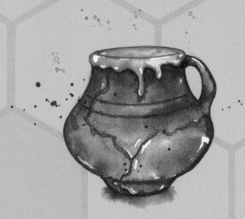

No other insect in existence has been more intently studied, experimented upon, worshipped and exploited than the humble honey bee. And the cause of it all has been what we get out of our relationship with that tiny creature – the sweet liquid that only a bee can produce, and which so delights human tastebuds that it has been described as the food of the gods: honey.

The origins of different foods are fascinating and complex, but nothing that we still put on our tables today can hold a candle to honey in terms of culinary history. Humans have been harvesting honey for nearly as long as we have existed, with records of the practice being documented in stone 8,000 years ago in the Cuevas de la Araña ('Spider Caves'), in Bicorp, Spain. The figure depicted on the cave wall is teetering precariously on a ladder, swiping honey from a wild bees' nest; that honey hunter would have suffered greatly for his or her prize. Incredibly, that same dangerous method is still in use today, though it is a swiftly dwindling tradition. Immense beehives high up on Himalayan cliffs in Nepal have, for centuries, inspired Gurung tribespeople to risk life and limb climbing rope ladders barefoot in order to cut off the honeycomb that is literally dripping over the sides of nests constructed within crevices.

DID YOU KNOW?

Honey is the only food humans eat
that is produced by an insect.

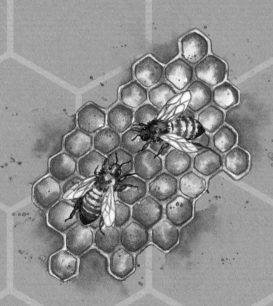

WHY ARE WE SO CRAZY ABOUT HONEY?

Humans are predisposed to crave sweetness in all its forms because sugar means energy, and energy means growth. From our mother's milk to our first teaspoon of honey, the best things in life are sweet!

For thousands of years, honey (from the Old English word 'hunig') would have been consumed in a very raw form – comb, brood and all – as it still is by some today. It wasn't until 1865 that a device was created to efficiently separate the honey from the comb. The centrifugal honey extractor, invented by Major Franz Elder von Hruschka, a Viennese who resided in Venice, signalled a huge development for beekeepers, allowing them to reuse the honeycomb and thereby maintain and grow their hives. Though there are several other methods still in use, the majority of commercial beekeepers today depend upon this invention.

The invention of the centrifugal extractor, along with wooden bee boxes with removable frames, allowed for the growth of commercial beekeeping, making honey harvesting a more profitable business.

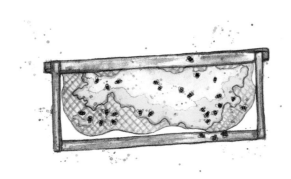

HONEY HARVESTING

Before turning to the honey, the beekeeper may harvest pollen, royal jelly and bee glue, or propolis, the resinous substance that bees create to keep their frames together. Propolis is prized for its medicinal qualities and can be sold separately or mixed with the honey. A special uncapping knife scrapes off the beeswax cappings (the plugs that bees use to seal the honeycomb), gathering them into a valuable and messy glob that can be processed for use in cosmetics, candles, polishes and art materials, among many other things. The frames are then spun in the extractor until most of the honey has been separated from the comb. After this, the beekeeper may choose to heat and filter the honey. Finally, the honey is funnelled into glass jars and taken to market, or to the beekeeper's kitchen.

Throughout history, bees have been kept not only for their honey, but also as a valuable source of beeswax, which had important medicinal, cosmetic and religious uses. Until 1900, only 100 per cent beeswax candles were allowed to be used in Catholic churches; even today, Church law requires that liturgical candles must contain a majority of beeswax.

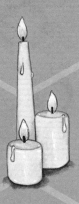

Busy as a Bee

It is clear from the description of this process that the beekeeper is merely a landlord: he or she provides housing for the bees, makes any necessary repairs, and collects rent once or twice a year. To understand what honey really is, we need to talk to the bees.

For a female worker bee, honey production is a very intimate matter. It is produced from her own body to be consumed as her only source of energy (along with pollen for protein) and as her invaluable contribution to the survival of the hive. During her short, intense lifespan of six weeks in the summer (five months in the winter), a worker bee will produce only one-twelfth of a teaspoon of honey. She does this by visiting (technically referred to as 'tapping') around 1,500 flowers a day. To produce half a kilo (1 pound) of honey, up to 2 million flowers must be tapped, requiring bees to fly around 50,000 miles.

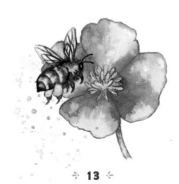

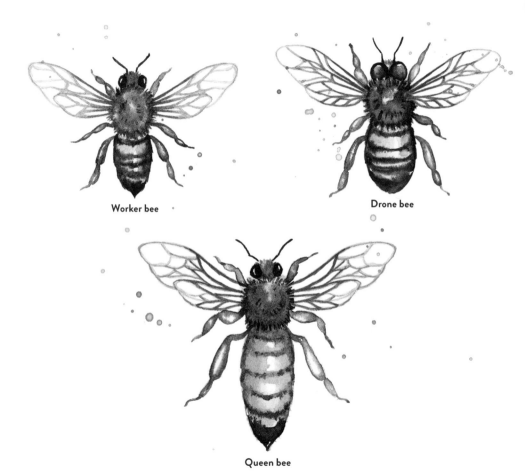

DID YOU KNOW?

Female worker bees are the only bees in the hive that produce honey. Queens only lay eggs, and drones only mate with the queen.

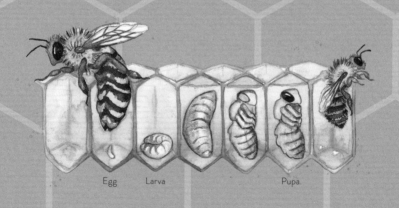

Egg　　Larva　　　　　Pupa

At twenty-one-days old, a worker bee will take her first foraging flight. Up to then, her 'house bee' duties have been the care and feeding of larvae, storing nectar and pollen, wax-comb building, hive defence and housekeeping. Finally, at middle age, she is able to stretch her wings and take flight as a 'field bee'.

Before the morning dew dries, the field bee sets off to work, collecting water, sap, nectar and pollen. When her ultraviolet vision locates a promising flower, the bee sits very still upon it or crawls inside it and sucks the nectar efficiently with her tongue. The nectar is stored inside the bee's honey sac (crop), an internal chamber in front of her honey stomach (ventriculus). The proventriculus between the two makes sure that no cross-contamination occurs. When the honey sac is full and she has also collected pollen in the pollen baskets on her hind legs, she makes a beeline for the hive.

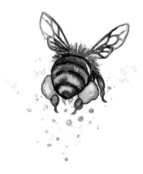

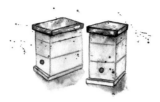

Turning Nectar to Honey

During the flight home, the nectar is already being broken down into glucose and fructose thanks to a protein enzyme in the honey stomach called invertase. When the field bee enters the hive, this is where the transformation from nectar to honey really begins, in curious and rather unappetizing ways. The field bee regurgitates the nectar and transfers it immediately to a house bee, tongue-to-tongue. Instinctively, the house bee deposits the nectar on the roof of a honey cell by regurgitation, where it will begin the drying process. Over the course of a few days, the nectar will be fanned by the wings of the house bees to bring the water content down from approximately 80 per cent to 18 per cent. By then most of the sucrose will have been broken down into glucose and fructose. When this is achieved, bees will cap the honey cells with wax produced by their glands, sealing out moisture so that the nectar will thicken as it ages. In this form, honey will remain edible indefinitely thanks to the stomach enzymes – glucose oxidase – that the bees contribute through regurgitation, and to the low moisture content. Glucose oxidase facilitates the production of hydrogen peroxide, which in turn provides honey's antimicrobial properties. Once that jar is unsealed, however, moisture could enter, causing fermentation.

Fermentation brings us to another use of honey: wine! The oldest wine in the world, which is still enjoyed today, is mead. Mead is simply fermented honey mixed with yeast and water and optional spices, fruits, grains or hops – the same basic recipe since its first recorded use in India 4,000 years ago. There are also written records of the enjoyment of mead in ancient Egypt, China, Minoa, Greece and Rome, as well as among the tribes of the Slavs, Celts and Germans. In several European countries in the Middle Ages, mead was the beverage of choice at wedding receptions, and a month-long (or the length of one moon cycle) supply of mead was given to newlyweds, giving rise to the expression 'honeymoon'.

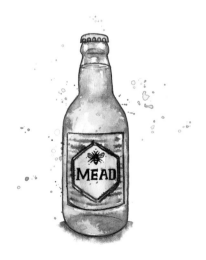

No wonder the ancients considered honey the food of the gods – it was a source of both sweetness and wine, not to mention its then-mysterious production. Some authors described how honey fell from the sky like the morning dew, and was collected from the upturned faces of the flowers by the bees, who then protected it in their hives as the gods' collaborators.

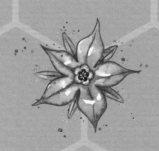

HONEY IN MYTHOLOGY AND FOLKLORE

Honey consumption was encouraged for virility and long life across cultures. The Greek gods Dionysus and Zeus were said to have been fed honey as babies, while at the opposite end of the scale, an extremely rare centenarian in ancient Rome, the philosopher Democritus, attributed his longevity to 'oil without and honey within'. Making the same claim, the Greek mathematician Pythagoras required his colleagues to consume honey as an energy-restorer after taxing work. Hippocrates, known as the father of modern medicine, prescribed honey mixed with hot water as a cure-all to his patients suffering from throat problems. This unaltered home remedy is now millennia old.

Traditional Ayurvedic medicine from India also describes honey as a cure-all, helping heal disordered digestion, skin, gums and teeth, the heart, the lungs, the eyes, and promote sleep. Avicenna, the Persian scientist of the Islamic Golden Age, gave this prescription: 'If you want to stay young, it is necessary to eat honey.' It makes sense at a very basic level: as honey is self-preserving, perhaps eating it could help preserve us as long as possible as well. While studies have yet to prove this for certain, countless honey-lovers have adopted this logic throughout the ages.

For all these reasons and many more, honey and bees feature predominantly in the records, mythology and folklore of ancient cultures across the world. The very earliest written records come from the Hittite Code, a Sumerian and Babylonian tablet of cuneiform writing from 2100 BC. The most well-known chronicle of honey and beekeeping comes from ancient Egypt, where bees were said to have been the very tears of Ra, god of the created world. Egyptians took bee worship and honey rituals to the highest level, bestowing the title of 'beekeeper' upon the pharaohs. Sacred animals were fed cakes sweetened with honey, while honey was also used in the mummification process and wax-sealed jars of it were found among the supplies prepared for the afterlife in royal tombs. And just as the Egyptians were preceded by the Sumerian civilization in their high regard for honey, subsequent civilizations imitated some of the practices of the Egyptian bee and honey worshipping society.

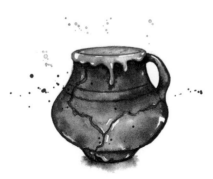

'When Ra weeps again, the water which flows from his eyes upon the ground turns into working bees. They work in flowers and trees of every kind and wax and honey come into being.'

Egyptian papyrus c. 300 BC

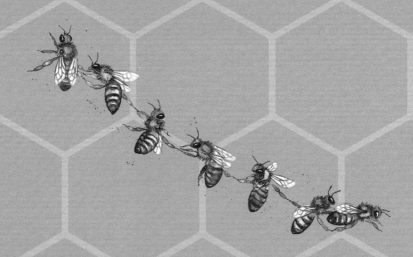

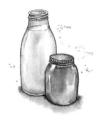

A Land Flowing with Milk and Honey

When the Israelites fled slavery in Egypt, it was to be led to a land 'flowing with milk and honey' (Exodus 33:3). Milk and honey were symbols not only of health and sweetness for body and soul, but also of a stable and peaceful society where cows, sheep and goats could be raised on abundant grazing lands, and colonies of bees could be kept and nourished by rich vegetation. To this day, 'the land of milk and honey' is used as a poetic expression describing a fertile utopia, overflowing with earthly goodness and beauty.

Because of its symbolic power of regeneration and blessings from the heavens, honey was offered in various forms to deities by all the cultures that used it. In the 12th century BC, records relate that Pharaoh Ramses III honoured the Nile god Hapi with fifteen tons of honey poured into the river. The Greeks and Romans offered jars of honey as well as honeycakes to their deities. In India still today, at the annual festival of Madhu, Buddhist monks are given gifts of honey by neighbours to mark the anniversary of Buddha's retreat to the forest, where he was given honey by monkeys for his sustenance.

Honey was also offered as payment or tribute to gain favour with other humans. Honeyed beer was used as a form of payment to workers, jars of honey were accepted as payment for taxes, and offered as tribute to conquering countries. Honey even appeared in marriage contracts. Egyptian grooms would commit to their brides with the following promise: 'I take you for my wife and bind myself to furnish you annually with twenty-four hins (14.5 kilos, or 32 pounds) of honey.' And in some European wedding customs, probably accompanied by the drinking of mead, the following toast was made, sometimes in the form of a song: 'Diligent is the life on a farm, like the life of the bee, and marriage is sweet as honey.'

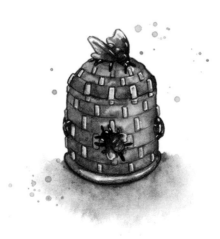

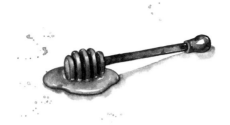

Mellified Man

Honey was considered to be life-giving by the ancients, and a tangible connection to the gods, which is perhaps why it was included in burial rituals, as a symbol of the afterlife. The most macabre folktale involving honey is that of the mellified man. Originating from Chinese tales called 'Chuogeng lu', or 'Talks While Resting the Plough' (c. 1366), the story goes that certain elderly men of Arabia would make living sacrifices of themselves by consuming no liquid or food, just honey, until their entire beings were saturated with it, even bathing exclusively in honey, and they subsequently died. Their bodies were then placed within a honey-filled stone coffin and transformed into human confections over the course of a century. Small amounts of the mellified man were then distributed for internal consumption for the treatment of wounds and fractures. Thankfully, the Chinese author of the tale concluded that the veracity of the account he received was dubious. Scholars believe that the story combines elements of the Assyrian and Egyptian practices of embalming the dead with the medicinal uses of honey, as well as a Burmese custom of preserving the bodies of high-level Buddhist monks in honey.

Sweet Endings

While the cautionary tale of the mellified man demonstrates that one can have too much of a good thing, the history of honey demonstrates that our love affair with the food of the gods has certainly withstood the test of time. And not only that, but it is experiencing a revival. The hope is that our society's increasing attraction to honey will provide the motivation we need to ensure the future of the honey bee and, by extension, 80 per cent of our cultivated crops pollinated by the creature. As an essential pollinator, the honey bee has long been the symbol of a flourishing ecology and civilization. Its demise signals our own. So, long live honey! Long live the honey bee! Long live life!

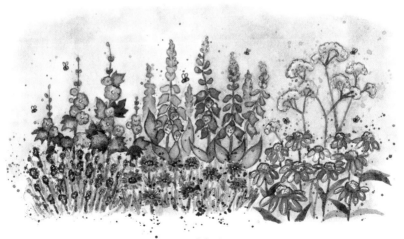

DID YOU KNOW?

Apis mellifera is the Latin nomenclature for honey bee, given to it by the Swedish botanist Carl Linnaeus in 1758. 'Mel' is Latin for honey, the Greek being 'μέλι/méli', and Hittite being 'mélit'.

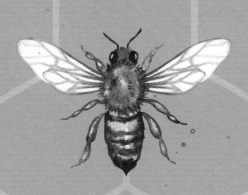

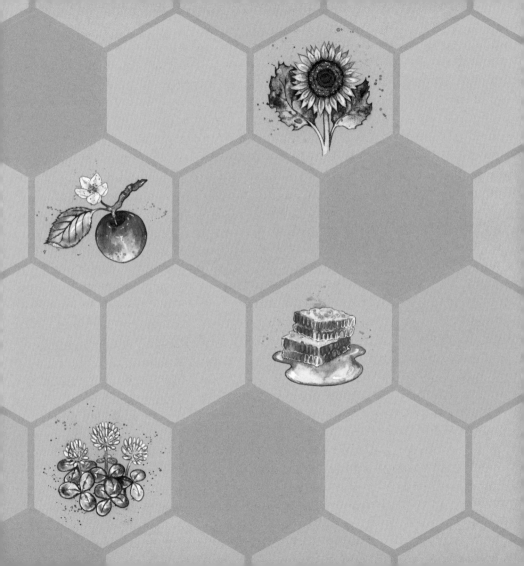

CHAPTER TWO

THE MANY SOURCES AND FLAVOURS OF HONEY

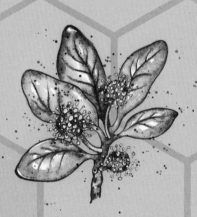

THE ABCs OF HONEY

One of the more interesting aspects of honey is the surprising array of flavours. Honey varies relatively little in terms of appearance or texture, and is made from only one ingredient: nectar. Yet there are more than 300 unique types of honey on the market today, each originating from a different flower source. Honey is found on every continent apart from Antarctica, and it is considered to be a valuable domestic and export product in most countries of the world. According to the United Nations Food and Agriculture Organization, China is the world's top producer of honey, New Zealand the top exporter, and the United States the top importer.

Naming Honey

Farmers' markets in Italy delighted me with their collection of varietals, and many hours were spent in sweet sampling. From the wet, Alpine north to the dry, sun-drenched islands of the south, Italy is uniquely positioned to produce what is referred to as artisan honey, created in the country's various microclimates. Some varieties of Italian honey even carry their own DOP (Denominazione di Origine Protetta/Protected Designation of Origin) label, designating them as products of a specific terroir, as is done with certain wines, cheeses and meats.

There are three basic categories of honey: single-origin, multi-flower and local. Single-origin honey comes mainly from the nectar of one specific plant, such as the orange blossom. Multi-flower comes from nectar collected from different plants. This may result in a varied flavour and appearance, and includes wildflower honey. Local honey is produced by nectar collected from a specific region or territory.

The flavour, consistency, colour, smell and medicinal properties of honey are dependent on the type of flower the nectar comes from. In most settings, bees collect nectar from a variety of sources and these combine to create a unique flavour profile that is different with every harvest.

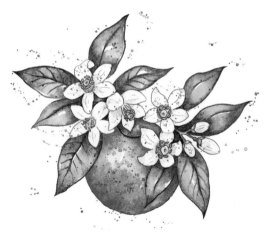

Depending on the location and time of year, there may be a dominant bloom that honey bees favour, and so their honey will be largely influenced by the properties of that nectar source. Beekeepers in different regions have learned to recognize local nectar sources and will label their honey as such. Examples include buckwheat honey, sage honey, tupelo honey, eucalyptus honey and heather honey.

Other beekeepers are more confident still in how they label their honey because they keep their bees on farms where only one type of crop is grown. In these vast agricultural settings, the bees are bound to make orange honey or avocado honey, for example, simply because nothing else is growing within the foraging range of bees (up to seven miles).

However, while it may sound appealing to consumers, most of the bees who yield varietal honey suffer undue stress from poor nutrition and exposure to pesticides. The safest way to buy honey is directly from a local beekeeper. Look for raw (unheated), minimally filtered honey, and avoid agricultural honeys made from a single crop. Honey is healthier for bees and humans when it comes from a more pristine, unaltered natural setting, with many flowers available to choose from. These honeys are sometimes called 'wildflower'.

FROM ACACIA TO WILDFLOWER: THE ALPHABET OF HONEY TYPES

Acacia honey is very sweet, with a clean, pure, classic flavour. It is made from the blossoms of the black locust tree in Europe and North America.

Alfalfa honey is light with a mild note and floral aroma. The vast alfalfa fields of North America produce the blue and purple blossoms bees love.

Apple blossom honey comes from large apple orchards after the bees pollinate the trees. It is light to medium amber in colour and contains a hint of apple flavour.

Aster honey is produced in the mid-south of the United States, from any of the flowers in the aster family. It is particularly sweet-smelling and prone to quick crystallization.

Avocado honey is gathered from California avocado blossoms. It is dark in colour, with a rich, buttery taste and a high level of vitamins and minerals.

Basswood honey is made from the basswood blossoms of North America, with a woodsy, minty taste and white hue.

Beechwood honey, also known as Honeydew honey, is rather unusual as it is sourced from the sap produced by aphids on the bark of the beechwood tree found on New Zealand's South Island. The sap is collected by the bees and converted into an aromatic and nutritious honey.

Blackberry honey is a light amber colour with a rich flavour, while still being light and fruity.

Blueberry honey has a slight tang and a fruity flavour. It is made in the United States in New England and Michigan from the tiny white flowers of the blueberry bush.

Buckwheat honey is sought after for its health benefits, as it is rich in iron and also tasty on toast. Its strong and spicy flavour makes it perfect for marinades. It is harvested in Canada and some northern states of the United States.

Carrot honey possesses an unusual combination of qualities: a smooth caramel flavour, a chocolatey aroma, a dark amber colour and a sharp, biting, earthy taste. Bees obtain nectar from wild carrots or when carrot plants run to seed.

Chestnut honey is strong, dark and slightly bitter. It pairs well with strong cheeses and dry red wine. Chestnut honey is harvested in Europe, Asia and the eastern United States.

Chinese tallow tree honey is a highly prized dark and tangy honey from the south-western United States into Texas.

Clover honey is classic honey that's light, sweet, floral and good in or on anything. Clover grows wild almost anywhere, making it an abundant nectar source for bees. Clover honey is harvested on five continents and is often creamed due to its rapid crystallization.

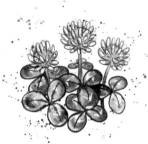

Coffee blossom honey is a rare product! Harvested from the fleeting blossoms of the coffee bush in Mexico and Guatemala, the honey tends to be dark, with a rich, deep flavour that matches its colour.

Eucalyptus honey, largely from Australia, has just a hint of menthol flavour to it, making it perfect for stirring into tea.

Fireweed honey has a markedly complex flavour and a slightly buttery texture. Like buckwheat honey, it can stand up to meats, marinades, glazes and grilling. It comes from a tall herb in the north-west United States.

Goldenrod honey is used to sweeten some biscuits and baked goods. It is produced in large quantities by bees after foraging the wild perennial in prairies, savannahs and meadows.

Heather honey is pungent and almost bitter, in a good way. It's great with smoky things, or on baked goods. Thick and amber, this honey packs a lot of protein. Heather honey has a long history in Great Britain and Germany, where it has been an essential ingredient in mead and liquors for millennia.

Lavender honey has the lovely aroma and delicate floral taste of the purple herb. It is produced largely in France and Spain.

Lehua honey is the only honey exclusively from Hawaii. Liquid upon harvest, it transforms into a creamy spread a few weeks later.

Linden honey is quite delicate and has a fresh, woodsy aroma that goes perfectly with a soothing tea at bedtime. This honey is harvested mainly in Denmark, from the small, yellowish-white flowers of the linden tree, and is touted for its medicinal benefits.

Macadamia honey has a distinctive sweet and nutty flavour with a lovely floral scent. It is largely harvested in Australia from the macadamia nut tree.

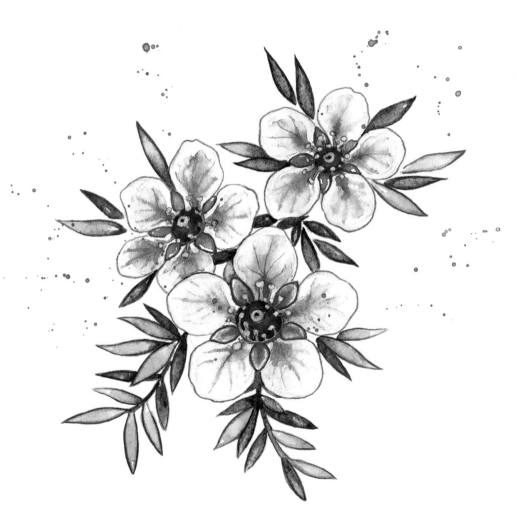

Manuka honey is made predominantly from the nectar of the manuka tree or tea tree, native to New Zealand and Australia. Although most honey has some medicinal value, manuka honey has elevated antibacterial properties that set it apart from other honeys. It is highly valued for its effectiveness in treating wounds, skin problems, cold symptoms and more.

Melipona honey, harvested from rare stingless bees, is revered in cultures where these species are native. It has been used as medicine by ancient peoples and was especially important in Mayan culture. In some countries, melipona honey is still used today and is particularly effective in treating eye conditions, such as cataracts. Melipona honey has a higher water content than that of European honey bees, but it does not ferment, suggesting a high level of antibacterial properties. Although more research needs to be done, some believe that melipona honey has unique and superior medicinal properties.

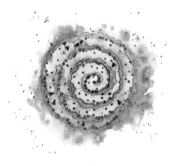

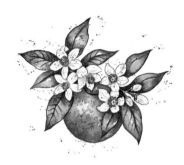

Mesquite honey is the ideal marinade if you are grilling over some smoky mesquite wood. Honey derived from the flowers of the mesquite tree has a smoky flavour, just like the wood.

Orange blossom honey is widely available, but watch out: much of the orange blossom honey on the market is artificially flavoured. Real orange blossom honey is mild and citrus-scented with a floral aroma, but it should not smell like perfume when you open the bottle. It is harvested in Florida and California.

Palmetto honey is a rare product from the saw palmetto tree in the southeast United States. It is robust and smoky.

Sage honey is similar to palmetto honey: mild, sweet and flexible. It is largely harvested in California and granulates slowly. For this reason, it is sometimes mixed in with other varietals to slow down crystallization.

Sourwood honey is caramel-like and buttery and delicious on toast, scones and muffins. It originates in the Appalachia region of the United States, from a late-season bloom of the sourwood tree.

Sunflower honey has a predictably floral scent and flavour, as it originates from the towering sunflower. As it crystallizes quickly, it is often consumed in this state as a spread.

Thyme honey is highly prized in Greece, where it must be made in small batches as it takes the bees four to five times as long to gather thyme honey than other local varietals, such as pine honey.

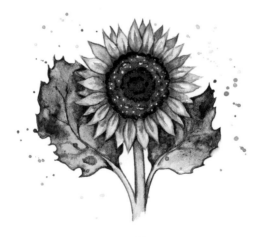

Tupelo honey is somehow sweeter than other types of honey but with a lovely, balanced, mild flavour. It is highly prized, often referred to as 'southern gold', and comes from the blossoms of tupelo trees that grow in swamps. It is resistant to crystallization due to its high fructose content.

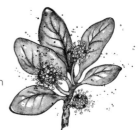

Ulmo honey is harvested in the forests of Argentina and Chile from the beautiful ulmo tree. It has medicinal qualities comparable to the more famous manuka honey, as well as a distinctive taste and aroma that has been described as reminiscent of almonds, cloves, vanilla, jasmine and aniseed.

Wildflower, or polyfloral, honey is light and fruity yet richly flavoured at the same time. The specific wildflowers from which the bees obtained the nectar to make this honey will make the flavour more delicate or intense. Wildflower honey is harvested all around the world.

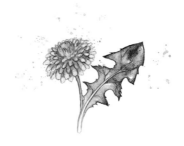

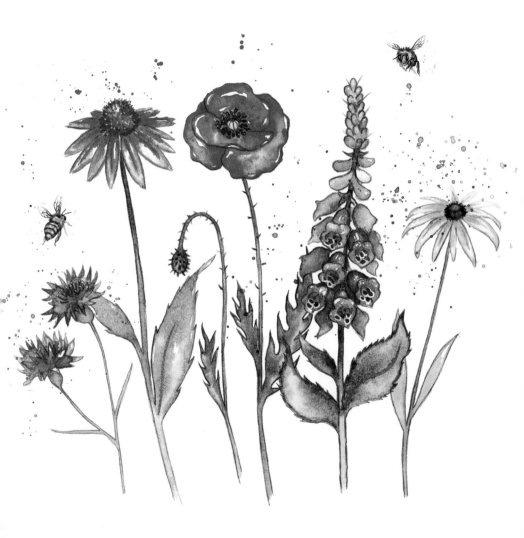

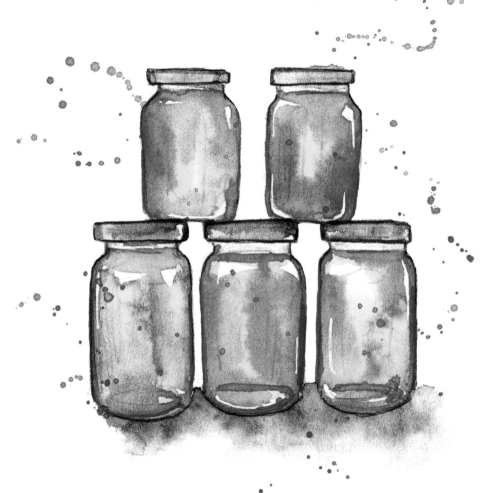

HONEY IN DIFFERENT FORMS

Honey can be distinguished by its production process. Most honey found in stores is in the 'liquid nectar' group, which comes as raw or pasteurized. Whipped honey is processed in such a way that it retains its sugar crystals and air is whipped in. This results in a smooth and spreadable texture. Finally, comb honey is a true speciality. It is sold in pieces and is felt to be a more 'natural' product with the minimum amount of production involved.

Some modern processing techniques involve heating the honey, which may diminish its well-documented medicinal benefits. The antimicrobial activity in most honey is connected to the levels of hydrogen peroxide produced by enzymes in the honey. When honey is heated, enzymes and other antibacterial components can be destroyed. For this reason, consumers should look for raw (unheated) honey.

Honey in Different Shades
There are different terms applied to the varying shades of honey. From palest to darkest, they are: white, white amber, amber, white subtle and dark.

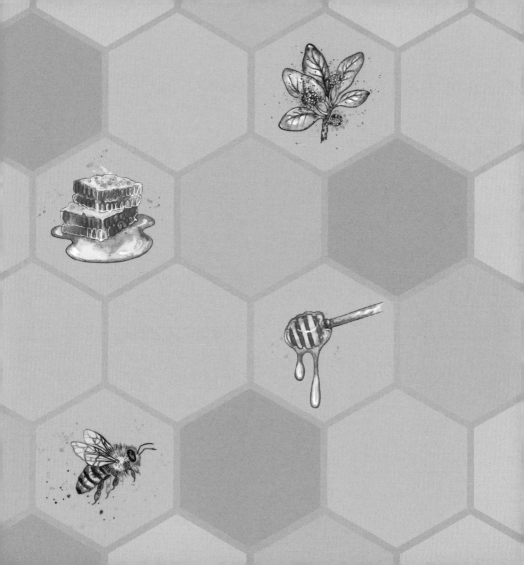

CHAPTER THREE

A HONEY BUYER'S GUIDE – HOW TO AVOID FOOL'S GOLD AND FIND THE REAL DEAL

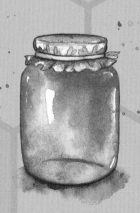

WHAT IS 'REAL' HONEY?

Quite simply, 'real' honey is produced only by honey bees; once anything else is added to it, it is no longer 100 per cent pure honey. Unfortunately, some of what passes for honey on the supermarket shelves does not meet this standard. All sorts of cheap fillers – not from a floral nectar source – are added to increase profits for producers and to lower the sale price. These include corn or rice syrup, sugar water, cane, beet or corn sugar, and even flour and starch. This adulterated honey is then either sold as is, or sold on to other companies, who mix the cheaper stuff into raw honey and sell it under their own 'mislabeled' label as genuine honey.

This unethical practice has a fitting name: 'honey laundering'. A series of developments preceded the honey laundering phenomenon, and it all began with trade issues. When high tariffs, known as 'anti-dumping' duties, were raised on cheap honey coming from China into the US, imports slowed. Shortly after that, Chinese beehives were devastated by foulbrood disease, and beekeepers fought back with animal antibiotics that were found to be carcinogenic. The FDA (US Food and Drug Administration) then banned Chinese honey altogether, and the flow of the sickening stuff ceased.

But before long, Chinese honey – both pure and tainted – found its way back into the US marketplace through intermediaries in other countries, who purchased, repackaged and 'transshipped' (moving cargo from one ship to another, rather than shipping directly) the honey to large honey importers in the US. In 2013, a company based in the US state of Michigan admitted to having purchased millions of dollars' worth of laundered honey and selling it under their own label.

The EU also banned imports of honey from China between 2002 and 2004 due to concerns over the use of antibiotics. And in 2019, the FSA (UK Food Standards Agency) warned again about the adulteration and impurity of honey in British supermarkets. Much of the honey sold in supermarkets is labelled 'Blend of EU/non-EU honeys', so it is impossible for the consumer to know where the product originated, and therefore how much is imported honey, where food safety requirements are lower than in the EU.

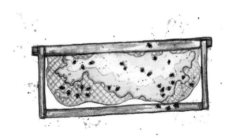

DID YOU KNOW?

'Honey laundering' is the unethical
practice of selling adulterated
honey under the guise of genuine honey.

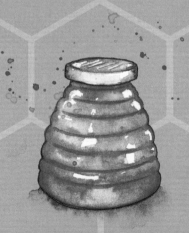

The Problem with Ultrafiltration

Another practice that corrupts the nutritious qualities of real honey is ultrafiltration. When honey is spun, dripped or spooned out of the honeycomb, along with it come all the bits and pieces that are not pure honey: bee body parts, pollen and wax. All are edible – and in the case of pollen, beneficial – but are not particularly attractive to consumers. So beekeepers strain the honey through a metal screen and a cloth to filter out these undesirables. This is the regular filtration process used by most beekeepers to package a clean-looking product. So far, so good.

Additional filtering of raw honey is referred to as ultrafiltration. The honey is diluted with water, filtered using charcoal, then filtered again through a membrane with a pore size of 0.45 micrometers using force from compressed air. Afterwards, the water is removed. The FDA calls this 'substantial transformation', because it so alters the natural identity of honey as to create a different kind of sweetener altogether. This type of watered-down sweetener is now in a more usable form, as an additive in beverages and cereals, which advertise that they are 'sweetened with honey'.

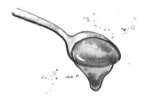

The majority of honey packers in the US say they do not subject their honey to ultrafiltration, but rather use a microfiltration system, which is USDA approved. This process uses filters with a pore size of 0.1 to 10 micrometers, which removes any particles visible to the naked eye. But why go to the trouble of filtering at all? It's all about aesthetics. To achieve 'Grade A' status under USDA regulations, honey must appear clear and possess a pleasing aroma and flavour.

Finely filtered honey will maintain a consistent, unblemished appearance, identical to all the other bottles on the shelf.

In the UK, honey that has undergone ultrafiltration, as opposed to the regular, approved filtration described above, must be labelled as 'filtered honey'.

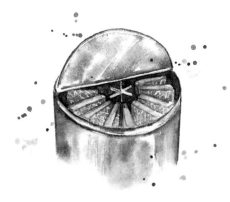

DID YOU KNOW?

Ultrafiltration removes much of what makes honey liquid gold in the first place: pollen, proteins and honey's natural antibacterial properties.

DID YOU KNOW?

Raw honey is almost straight from the hive, bee bits and all. Unpasteurized honey is slightly filtered and heated. Pasteurized honey is heated to 70°C (160°F) to slow down crystallization and resist granulation.

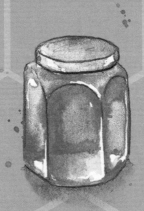

The Problem with Pasteurization

Similar to the aesthetic requirement of filtration, honey heated to 70°C (160°F) is unlikely to ever crystallize, keeping it in its perfect liquid state on supermarket shelves indefinitely. Yet many consumers today are still unaware that crystallization is a normal and harmless process that honey goes through with time and colder temperatures, and that it can be restored to a liquid state through immersion in a warm-water bath. And honey sellers aren't going to take the risk that buyers possess this knowledge; they are simply going to heat their honey to 70°C (160°F).

The problem with heating to the level of pasteurization is that the honey will then possess few antioxidants, amino acids, vitamins, minerals and healthy enzymes, effectively becoming an expensive form of sugar. And as pasteurization does not kill botulism spores, there are no safety benefits to the treatment.

Heating honey slightly, keeping it below the pasteurization temperature point to maintain the nutritional integrity, is a common beekeeping practice to decrease viscosity in order to aid in the bottling process. This type of honey is called 'unpasteurized' and is slightly filtered, as distinguished from raw honey, which is neither filtered nor heated.

Good Stuff In, Good Stuff Out

Honey is a unique agricultural product, as beekeepers cannot control what their bees feed upon in the same way that farmers can control the diet of their livestock. The only way beekeepers can guarantee that the honey they are selling is truly organic is to provide enough pesticide-free foraging land within the typical flight range of the bee. Bees usually find the pollen and water they need within three miles of the hive, but will fly up to seven miles or more if necessary. To restrict the bees' foraging range, and therefore potential exposure to pesticides, beekeepers interested in selling organic honey must immerse their hives in a rich, organic foraging environment. Bees are famously efficient and will not fly any further than necessary. Uncultivated prairies, conservation land and forests are the safest bets for hive placement in order to harvest premium organic honey.

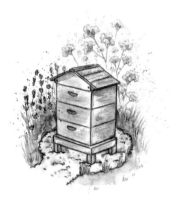

DID YOU KNOW?

A clean environment produces clean honey. Bees will feed upon nutrient-rich, organic sources of nectar if that is what is proximate to their hive.

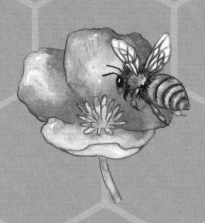

DID YOU KNOW?

Melissopalynology is the science of pollen analysis in honey, which provides its botanical and geographical origin, as well as other potential information, such as how the honey was extracted and if it has been contaminated by any metals or additives.

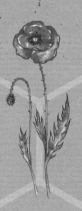

Putting Your Jar to the Test

How can a consumer be sure they've hit the jackpot and that their honey is the real deal? There are several tests you can subject your honey to in order to uncover its true identity. These include plopping it in water to see if it dissolves, setting it on fire, smearing it on bread, or just putting it on your thumb to see if it slides off. Unfortunately, the chemical make-up of honey is not that easy to determine. So, if you don't have a melissopalynology lab in your basement, you're better off putting your local beekeeper to the test.

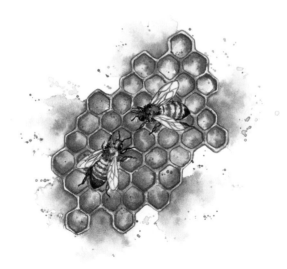

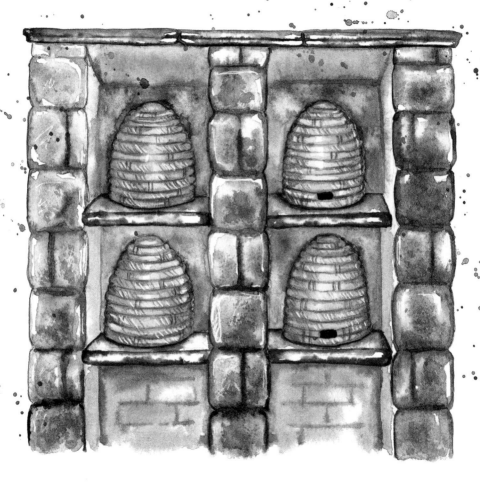

Befriend a Beekeeper
To get honey in its purest and most nutritious form, it pays to go straight to the source. If you don't keep your own bees, there are plenty of amateur and professional beekeepers around, who can be found through an online search or at local farmers' markets. Knowing the beekeeper personally means you can discover the type of natural environment in which the beehives are placed, whether the bees' diet is supplemented at all, and what sort of heating and filtration process the beekeeper uses during bottling.

The next step away from this is to always buy honey that is labelled raw or unpasteurized and 'true source certified'. Primarily based in the US, the True Source Honey programme is a voluntary organization for beekeepers, packers, importers and exporters. It certifies that the honey carrying their label has been ethically sourced and its origin verified. This in turn means the honey has been minimally filtered and the pollen is still present. The research of a similar organization, the International Honey Commission, contributed to the creation of the EU Honey Directive, an effort to create quality standards and transparent labelling of honey within the EU. Also in the UK, the London Honey Awards encourages the production of high-quality honey through competitions and awards, as well as a honey sommelier certification course. Pollen is just an accidental byproduct that ends up in honey because bees carry it with them to the hive after harvesting floral nectar. However, it comes in handy for humans as the only way to trace the location of the original flower or plant that helped create the particular jar of honey you are consuming.

If you are interested in getting a daily dose of local pollen to naturally build immunity to seasonal allergies, be sure to buy local honey harvested during the season when you most experience allergic symptoms.

Finally, you will want to have a quick glance at the label to be sure there is only one thing listed in the ingredients section: honey! Manufacturers could include flavours, spices, fruit and so on, which might introduce artificial sweeteners into the mix. Instead, you could experiment with additions at home and create a uniquely customized honey that would make a delicious handcrafted gift, or as something to proudly pull out as you pour a visitor a cup of tea.

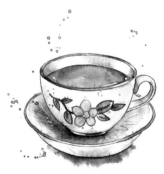

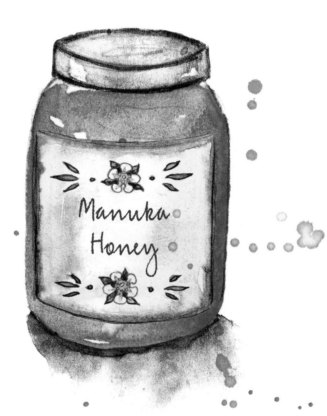

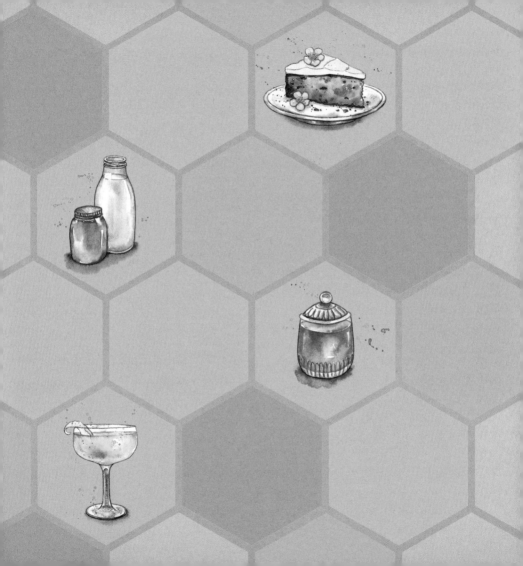

CHAPTER FOUR

FOOD AND DRINK RECIPES WITH HONEY

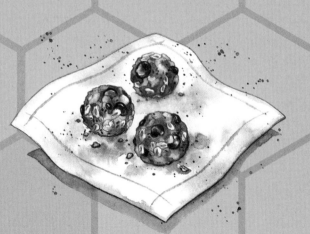

Of course, good-quality honey should be enjoyed straight from the jar, savouring its particular flavour and texture on the tip of the tongue. But if you'd like to enrich your dishes and beverages with the mellow, healthy sweetness of honey, here are a few delicious recipes using this 'nectar of the gods'.

Honey Syrup

To make honey syrup, combine equal amounts of honey and water in a saucepan and dissolve over a low heat while stirring. Allow to cool then transfer to a glass jar and refrigerate until chilled, about 2 hours. Store covered in the fridge for up to 1 week.

Please note: Be sure to always follow all the steps in the recipes carefully, leave hot liquids to cool and take care not to cause injury on sharp knives or to burn yourself while cooking. Read safety instructions on any items used and follow manufacturer's guidelines and safety precautions. Examine the contents of ingredients prior to preparation and consumption to be fully aware of the presence of substances that might provoke an adverse reaction in some consumers.

Family-friendly Beverages

HONEY-GINGER LEMONADE PUNCH

This delicious recipe is inspired by the National Honey Board and takes lemonade to a new level. For extra variety, you can substitute sparkling water for the water in the lemonade.

Makes around 2.5 litres (4½ pints)

For the honey-ginger syrup
340g (12oz) honey
5 thin slices of fresh root ginger, peeled
125ml (4fl oz) water

For the lemonade
250ml (8fl oz) freshly squeezed lemon juice
700ml (1¼ pints) apple juice
1.25 litres (2¼ pints) water
Lemon slices, to garnish

1. Simmer the honey-ginger syrup ingredients in a heavy saucepan for about 30 minutes, then set aside to cool. Remove the ginger slices and discard.
2. In a large jug, combine the lemon juice, apple juice and water. Stir in the cooled syrup.
3. Fill each glass with ice and the punch, and garnish with a lemon slice.

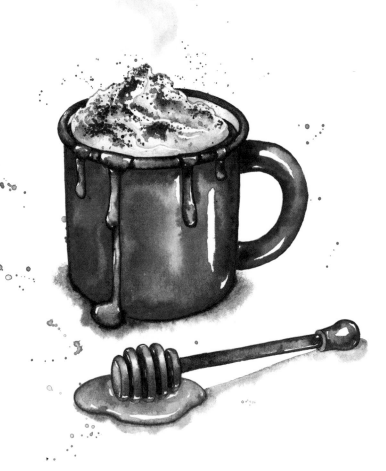

MAYA'S HONEYED HOT COCOA

This is my daughter's own recipe, which she serves on cold nights as a special family treat, or to earn points with kids when babysitting!

Serves 3–4 (depending on mug size)

810ml (1½ pints/3¼ cups) whole milk
1½ tsp unsalted butter
4 tsp double cream
½ tsp vanilla extract
1½ tsp freshly-ground coffee (optional – for an adult-only version!)
Pinch of salt
Pinch of ground cinnamon
Pinch of ground nutmeg, plus extra for garnish (optional)
Pinch of ground ginger
Pinch of ground allspice
1 tbsp smooth peanut butter
4 tsp cocoa powder
3 tbsp honey
Whipped cream, to serve

continued

1. Warm the milk in a pan over a low heat. Add the butter, cream, vanilla extract, coffee (if using), salt and spices and whisk until smooth. Turn off the heat.
2. In a separate pan, blend the peanut butter with a little of the milk mixture over a low heat until smooth. Continue to add the remaining milk mixture, stirring constantly. Blend in the cocoa powder until smooth, then blend in the honey and heat until hot. Allow to cool for as long as necessary until of suitable drinking temperature.
3. Pour into large mugs and top with whipped cream and a dusting of nutmeg, if desired, and serve.

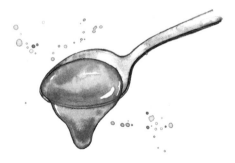

FRUIT SMOOTHIE

Honey is not only the perfect natural sweetener, but also a health- and energy-boosting ingredient for your morning or snack-time smoothie. The thick, rich texture of honey adds bulk to the mix and makes it palatable to the toddlers and other sweet-toothed members of your household who otherwise might balk at health drinks. Any combination of honey, fruit/berries, leafy greens, dairy/dairy alternative and supplements can work; here's a particularly tasty and hearty combination of ingredients. Add cold water as needed to thin the smoothie to your desired consistency.

Serves 2

285g (10oz) Greek yogurt
45g (1½oz) rolled oats
85g (3oz) honey
190ml (6½fl oz) almond or oat milk

140g (5oz) frozen berries of choice (we like strawberries in this recipe)
140g (5oz) frozen peaches or bananas

1 Combine all the ingredients in a blender and pulse until the fruit is broken up a bit, then blend on high until all the ingredients are smooth. Pour into glasses and serve immediately.

Cocktails and Alcoholic Elixirs

GOLD RUSH

If you prefer bourbon or whisky to gin, try this recipe, which is similar to The Bee's Knees.

Serves 1

60ml (2fl oz) bourbon
22ml (¾fl oz) fresh lemon juice
22ml (¾fl oz) Honey Syrup (see page 66)

1 In a cocktail shaker, combine all three ingredients, shake vigorously and strain into a rocks glass with a large ice cube.

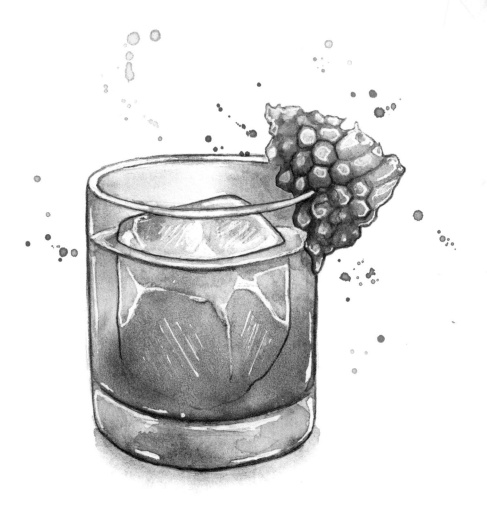

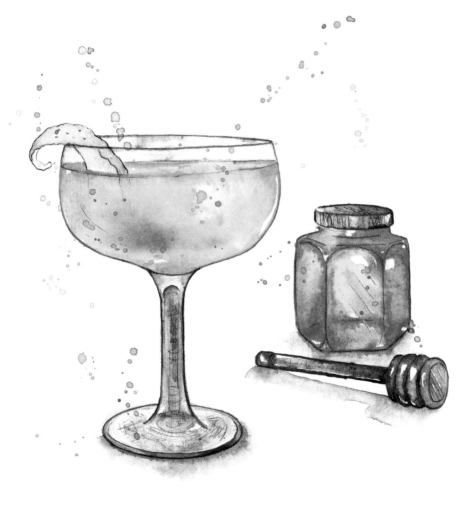

THE BEE'S KNEES

The Bee's Knees cocktail is delicious in its simplicity – but don't let that fool you. To be the ultimate bee's brew means using the very best ingredients. Fortunately, there are only three: gin, honey and lemon. Invented during the Prohibition era, The Bee's Knees has gone through a bit of a renaissance in the twenty-first century. Today's mixologists love a good experiment, and here the drink's profile can change considerably depending on gin style and honey type. So go on, why not create your own home mixology lab!

Serves 1

45ml (1½fl oz) gin
15ml (½fl oz) Honey Syrup
 (see page 66)
15ml (½fl oz) freshly squeezed
 lemon juice
Lemon zest or honeycomb, to serve

continued

1. Add 3–4 ice cubes to a cocktail shaker. Pour in all three ingredients and shake well. Strain into a chilled coupe glass.
2. Serve with a twist of lemon zest or, if you're feeling daring, a shred of honeycomb, and enjoy!

Note: A traditional London dry gin will provide a more floral, juniper-enhanced flavour. Old Tom gin adds a sweet citrus flavour that can be balanced with a floral honey.

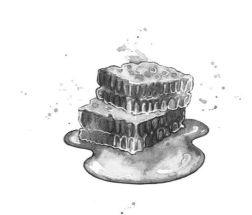

SPICED HOT HONEY TODDY

My dad acquired the habit of sipping a hot toddy on rainy nights during his years in Scotland, and he rarely caught a cold. It was his speciality whenever my mother had a sore throat. Here's a particularly effective and spicy recipe inspired by the National Honey Board website, created by mixologist Julia Momose.

Serves 1

½ tsp whole allspice
½ tsp whole pink peppercorns
½ tsp ground cinnamon, plus an extra cinnamon stick to garnish (optional)

375ml (13fl oz) water
1 tsp chamomile flowers, or 1 chamomile tea bag
2 tsp honey (preferably buckwheat)
45ml (1½fl oz) rum

continued

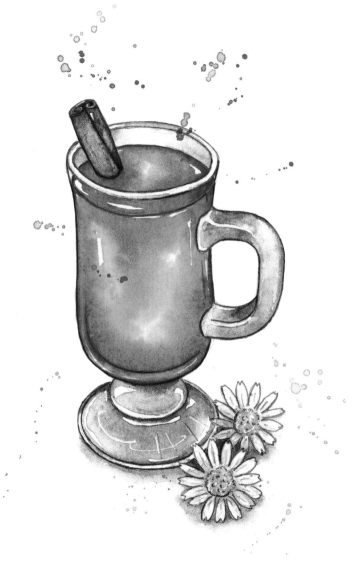

1. Lightly crack the spices using a pestle and mortar, or on a cutting board by tapping with the end of a rolling pin.
2. Toast the spices in a dry frying pan over a low heat until aromatic, about 2–3 minutes.
3. Pour the water directly into the pan over the toasted spices and bring to a simmer over a medium heat. Simmer for 5 minutes.
4. Turn off the heat, add the chamomile flowers or tea bag and steep for 5 minutes.
5. Combine the honey and rum in a mug.
6. Strain the spiced chamomile tea into the mug and stir to combine. Garnish with a cinnamon stick, if desired.

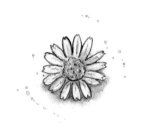

Coffee and Tea

Honey is far superior to sugar as a sweetener in coffee and tea, for taste, texture and health benefits. Once your tastebuds have become accustomed to its natural, more mellow sweetness, sugar will suddenly seem sickly by comparison. Honey also slightly thickens beverages, making it an ideal ingredient in coffee and tea recipes.

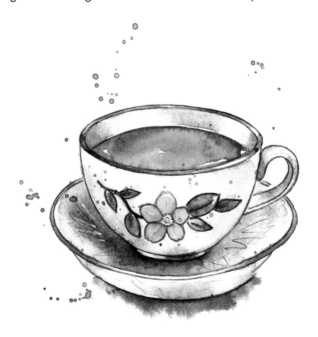

TONY'S CRAZY TEA

One Thanksgiving weekend years ago, our entire household of visitors came down with a miserable cold. My husband Tony served us this strange brew constantly, keeping us healthy and energetic throughout the festivities. Our friends dubbed it 'Tony's Crazy Tea' and ended up recreating it and selling it to adventurous patrons at their New York shawarma joint!

Serves 1

Quantities below are all according to individual taste and how strong you like your flavours.

Freshly chopped garlic
Lemon slices, reserving one slice to garnish
Fresh mint, reserving one sprig to garnish
Honey

1. Combine the freshly chopped garlic, lemon slices, fresh mint, and honey to taste in a pan with 1 litre (1¾ pints or 34fl oz) of water, and boil until it reaches your desired consistency and quantity.
2. Garnish the cup with a sprig of fresh mint or a slice of lemon.

CAFÉ MIEL

This recipe calls for a scrumptious spiced honey syrup, which you can whip up ahead of time and keep on hand to transform your espresso into a barista-level brew.

Serves 2

For the spiced honey syrup
240ml (8fl oz) Honey Syrup (see page 66)
⅛ tsp ground cardamom
¼ tsp ground ginger
¼ tsp ground cinnamon, plus extra to dust

2 double shots of espresso
Steamed whole milk, to taste

1. For the spiced honey syrup, whisk all the ingredients together. Bottle and set aside. Shake before use.
2. Combine 90ml (3fl oz) spiced honey syrup and a double shot of espresso in each glass mug.
3. Top with steamed milk, to taste. Lightly dust the foam with cinnamon.

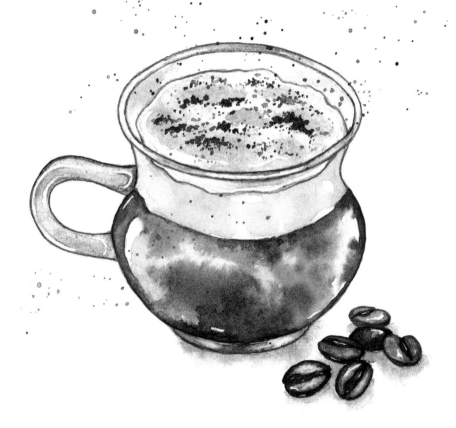

Appetizers

GOAT'S CHEESE, HONEY AND FRUIT CROSTINI

These three ingredients are natural partners atop crispy slices of baguette, and extremely simple to prepare for an elegant start to a honey-infused feast, or as a light nibble alongside your honeyed cocktails.

Serves 3–4 as an appetiser (or 1 as an indulgent lunch!)

1 baguette, thinly sliced (into 2-cm/¾-inch slices)
225g (8oz) creamy goat's cheese, thinly sliced
2 tbsp honey, plus extra to drizzle

250g (9oz or approximately 2 cups) thinly sliced fruit of your choosing (strawberries, peaches, pears or blackberries)

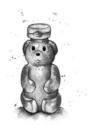

1. Preheat the oven to 180°C (350°F) and spread the bread slices over a baking sheet. Bake for 10 minutes or until slightly crispy.
2. Combine the goat's cheese and honey until smooth and spread over each slice of bread. Top with the fruit and drizzle with extra honey.

> **Note:** To prepare in advance, toast the bread and spread with the cheese and honey, then store in an airtight container in the fridge overnight. Just before serving, top with the fruit and drizzled honey.

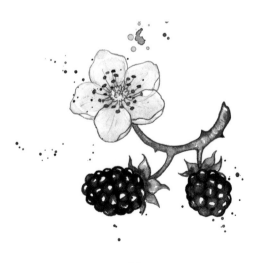

PROSCIUTTO HONEY WRAPS

Warm peaches, prosciutto, honey and goat's cheese is a delectable combination. This recipe makes an elegant appetizer for outdoor summertime gatherings.

Makes 12

1 large peach (fresh or tinned)
2½ tsp honey
½ tsp butter, melted
6 tbsp goat's cheese

45g (1½oz) baby spinach, loosely packed
4 slices prosciutto

1. Cut the peach in half and remove the stone (if using a fresh peach).
2. Combine ½ tsp honey with the butter and brush the peach halves lightly with the mixture.
3. Heat an outdoor barbecue or indoor grill on a low–medium heat and place both halves onto the grill or pan. Cook for about 2 minutes on each side, or until lightly charred but still firm.
4. Cut the peach halves into 1-cm (½-inch) slices (about 12) or drain 12 slices if using tinned.
5. Put 1½ tsp goat's cheese on each peach slice and place on top of 4 baby spinach leaves.

6. Slice the prosciutto lengthways to create 12 strips. Wrap the centre of each peach/cheese/spinach bundle with a prosciutto strip.
7. Arrange on a serving platter and drizzle each bundle with a little of the remaining honey.

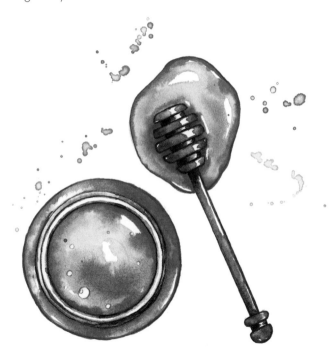

Salad Dressings and Sauces

HONEY-SOY SALAD DRESSING

This Asian-flavoured recipe can be used as a salad dressing or drizzle over meat, poultry or fish.

Makes enough for 1–2 salads

½ tsp honey
1 tbsp very hot water
2 tsp apple cider vinegar

1 tsp soy sauce
1 tbsp sherry vinegar

1. Put the honey and hot water in a jar and shake vigorously. Add the other ingredients and mix well.

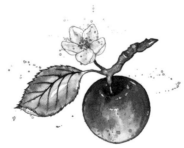

HONEY-LEMON DRESSING

This simple dressing brings flavour to any salad or chicken dish.

Makes enough for 1–2 salads

1 tbsp olive oil
2 tsp lemon juice
1 tsp honey

Pinch of dried oregano (or ½ tsp finely chopped fresh)

1. Combine the ingredients together in a small container. Set aside until ready to use.

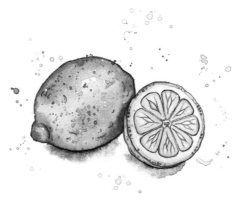

VERSATILE HONEY-MUSTARD SAUCE

Almost any food would benefit from being topped with, dipped into or marinated in this easy-peasy sauce. Try it with chicken, fish, meatballs or potatoes.

Makes enough for 1–2 portions

115g (½ cup) mayonnaise
1 tbsp Dijon-style mustard
3 tbsp honey

1. In a medium bowl, combine all the ingredients together. Chill in the fridge for at least 2 hours before serving.

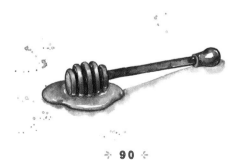

Poultry, Meat, Seafood and Fish Dishes

HONEY-LIME CHICKEN SKEWERS

This is another easy summertime recipe. These skewers would be a filling appetizer paired with one of the honeyed cocktails.

Serves 8

2 tbsp honey
3 tbsp soy sauce
1 tbsp olive oil

Juice of 1 lime
450g (1lb) skinless, boneless chicken breast strips

1. In a small bowl, whisk all the liquid ingredients together until completely blended. Pour the mixture into a freezer bag and add the chicken strips. Reseal the bag and gently shake to cover the chicken strips. Allow to marinate for 2 hours.
2. If using wooden skewers, soak them in water for 15 minutes. Preheat the grill to medium–high.
3. Remove the chicken strips from the marinade and thread onto the skewers. Grill for 8 minutes, turning occasionally, or until the juices are clear and the chicken is fully cooked.

STOUT AND HONEY BEEF ROAST

This recipe will keep you warm and cosy. The dish is best paired with a pint of creamy stout and a roaring fire.

Serves 12

12 small red potatoes, scrubbed
6–7 medium carrots, peeled and cut into 1-cm (½-inch) pieces
2 medium onions, quartered
1.8kg (4lb) braising steak
400ml (14fl oz) beef stock
250ml (8fl oz) dark ale or stout (or use additional beef stock)
170g (6oz) honey
3 garlic cloves, crushed
1 tsp dried marjoram
1 tsp dried thyme
½ tsp salt
½ tsp pepper
¼ tsp ground cinnamon
2 tbsp cornflour
60ml (2fl oz) cold water
Finely chopped fresh thyme (optional)

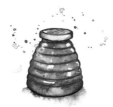

1. Place the potatoes, carrots and onions in a slow cooker with the beef. Combine the stock, beer, honey, garlic, marjoram, thyme, salt, pepper and cinnamon in a small bowl, then pour over the beef and vegetables. Cook, covered, on low for 8–10 hours until the meat and vegetables are tender.
2. Remove the beef from the slow cooker using a slotted spoon and set aside. Strain the cooking juices, reserving the vegetables and 250ml (8fl oz) liquid. Skim the fat from the reserved liquid, and transfer the liquid to a small saucepan. Bring to the boil.
3. Combine the cornflour and cold water until smooth, then gradually stir into the juices in the pan. Return to the boil and stir until thickened, about 2 minutes. Serve with the beef and vegetables, garnished with fresh thyme, if desired.

Note: If you do not have a slow cooker, you can instead cook this in the oven at 160°C (325°F) for 3 hours.

HONEY-GARLIC PORK CHOPS

The sweet and savoury combination in this glaze is a delicious complement for pork, but would also work well as a glaze for chicken and potatoes, or as a dipping sauce.

Serves 6

120g (4¼oz) ketchup
2⅔ tbsp honey
2 tbsp low-sodium soy sauce

2 garlic cloves, crushed
6 × 110g (4oz) pork chops

1. Preheat the grill to medium.
2. Whisk the ketchup, honey, soy sauce and garlic together in a bowl to make a glaze.
3. Cook the pork chops on both sides under the preheated grill or on a barbecue. Lightly brush the glaze onto each side of the chops as they cook; grill until no longer pink in the centre, about 7–9 minutes per side. A cooking thermometer inserted into the centre should read 63°C (145°F).

HONEY HADDOCK

Honey complements all kinds of fish. This recipe was included for its simplicity and crunch.

Serves 6

170g (6oz) butter
225g (8oz) buttery crackers, crushed (such as RITZ Crackers)
680g (1½lb) haddock, patted dry
170g (6oz) honey
1 tsp dried parsley

1. Preheat the oven to 200°C (400°F).
2. Melt two-thirds of the butter in a pan, then remove from the heat and mix the crushed crackers into the melted butter.
3. Place the haddock in a shallow baking dish and cover with the butter-cracker mixture.
4. Bake the haddock for around 25 minutes, until the flesh flakes easily with a fork.
5. Melt the remaining butter and stir through the honey and parsley until blended.
6. Drizzle the honey butter over the cooked haddock and return to the oven for 5 minutes or so, until the top is browned.

HONEY-BRINED GRILLED PRAWNS

In this recipe, the prawns receive a triple treatment of honey: coated, tossed and drizzled.

Serves 6

- 680g (1½lb) unpeeled large prawns
- 250ml (8fl oz) boiling water
- 2 tbsp cooking salt
- 5 tbsp wildflower honey
- 16 ice cubes
- 3 tbsp red wine vinegar
- 60ml (2fl oz) extra-virgin olive oil
- 15g (½oz) finely chopped fresh flat-leaf parsley
- 3 tbsp finely chopped white onion
- 2 tbsp finely chopped fresh oregano
- 2 garlic cloves, crushed
- Cooking oil spray
- 1 small red chilli, thinly sliced

1. Devein the prawns, and remove the legs from the shells, if desired (do not remove the shells).
2. Combine the boiling water, salt and half the honey in a large bowl, and stir until the salt dissolves. Add the ice cubes and stir until the mixture cools. Add the prawns and refrigerate for 20 minutes.

3. Remove the prawns from the bowl, discarding the liquid. Pat the prawns dry with paper towels and toss in a bowl with 1½ tsp honey.
4. Preheat the grill to medium–high, or alternatively use a griddle pan on the stove.
5. Place the red wine vinegar and remaining honey in a large bowl; stir with a whisk to combine. Gradually add the olive oil, stirring constantly with the whisk until well blended. Stir in the parsley, onion, oregano and garlic.
6. Arrange the unpeeled prawns on the grill or griddle coated with cooking spray. Cook the prawns, uncovered, for 2½ minutes on each side, or until lightly charred and cooked through. Add the prawns to the bowl with the vinegar mixture and toss well to coat.
7. Arrange the prawns on a platter and top with the sliced chilli.

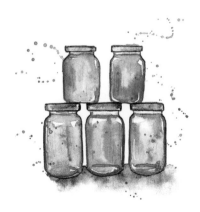

Desserts and Sweet Snacks

Tip: You can substitute honey for white sugar in any dessert recipe. If the recipe calls for more than 200g (7oz) sugar, reduce any other liquids in the recipe by 60ml (2fl oz), if substituting with honey. Some scrumptious experimentation may be necessary. If honey causes your baked desserts to brown too quickly, try lowering the oven temperature slightly.

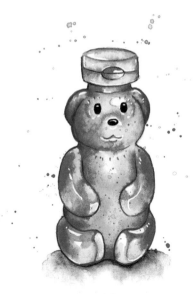

NO-BAKE HONEY ENERGY BITES

A honey-sweetened snack that still tastes like a treat but provides much better fuel for both body and brain.

Makes 15

75g (2¾oz) peanuts, finely chopped
135g (4¾oz) oats
50g (1¾oz) flax seeds
55g (2oz) almond flour
3 tbsp unsweetened cocoa powder

2 tbsp peanut butter powder
110g (4oz) mini chocolate chips (optional), divided
120g (4¼oz) peanut butter
110g (4oz) honey
2 tbsp almond or soy milk

1   Line a baking tray with parchment paper. Place the chopped peanuts in a small bowl and set aside.
2   In a food processor, combine two-thirds of the oats with the flax seeds, almond flour, cocoa powder, peanut butter powder and half the chocolate chips if using. Pulse several times until it resembles coarse meal.

continued

3. Add the peanut butter, honey and almond or soy milk to the oat mixture and process until the mixture comes together.
4. Transfer the oat mixture to a large bowl and mix in the remaining oats and chocolate chips, if using – your hands work best for this!
5. Scoop out 2.5-cm (1-inch) clusters of the mixture and roll into about 15 balls with your hands. Then dip the bites in the finely chopped peanuts. Place each ball on the baking tray and chill in the fridge until firm.
6. When the bites are chilled and set, store in an airtight container for up to a week.

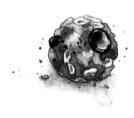

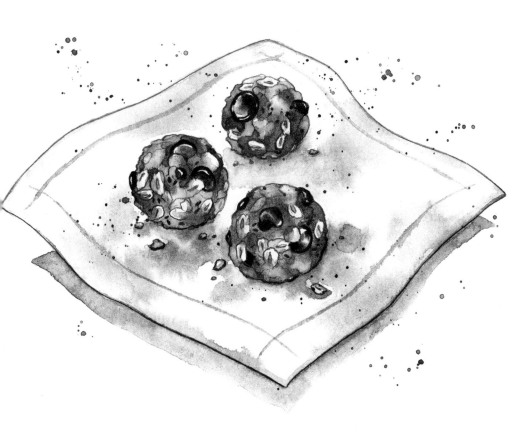

HONEY CAKE WITH HONEY BUTTERCREAM ICING

Here's a sunny option for a birthday cake that will sweeten up your party.

Serves 8

For the honey cake
140g (5oz) butter
255g (9oz) honey
85g (3oz) light soft brown sugar
1 tbsp water
2 eggs, beaten
245g (8½oz) self-raising flour
1 tsp ground cinnamon

For the icing
110g (4oz) butter
200g (7oz) icing sugar
1 tbsp honey

1 Preheat the oven to 180°C (350°F). Grease a 20-cm (8-inch) cake tin.
2 Put the butter, honey, sugar and water into a saucepan over a low heat, stirring occasionally, until the butter has melted.
3 Remove from the heat and stir in the eggs, flour and cinnamon; give the mixture a quick whisk to remove any lumps.
4 Pour the mixture into the cake tin and bake for 40–45 minutes, until a skewer inserted into the centre comes out clean.

5   Leave the cake in the tin for 5 minutes before transferring to a cooling rack.
6   To make the icing, cream together the butter and sugar until light and fluffy, then stir in the honey.
7   Once the cake has cooled, spread a generous layer of icing across the top (and the sides, if desired). Serve and enjoy!

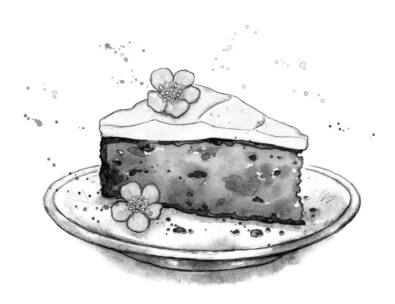

APPLE BAKLAVA BITES

I've saved the best for last. It is my personal opinion that baklava is the best use of honey. Here is a (slightly) healthier and easier variation on the classic Middle Eastern treat, compliments of the National Honey Board.

Makes 15

1 packet mini filo shells (15 shells)
55g (2oz) walnut pieces, chopped
1 tbsp butter, cut into 8 cubes
1 tbsp caster sugar
½ tsp ground cinnamon
2 drops vanilla extract
Pinch of salt

1 apple, peeled and finely diced
1 tbsp plain flour
60ml (2fl oz) water
85g (3oz) honey
Large pinch of ground cardamom (optional)
Juice of ½ lemon

1. Preheat the oven to 180°C (350°F). Arrange the filo shells on a baking sheet.
2. Place the walnuts, butter, sugar, cinnamon, vanilla extract and salt in a food processor or blender, and process until the ingredients come together into a chunky dough.

3. Combine the apple and flour in a medium mixing bowl. Add the walnut mixture and mix well.
4. Pack about 1 heaped teaspoon of the apple–walnut mixture into each filo shell and bake for 10 minutes.
5. While the baklava bake, combine the water and honey in a saucepan. Bring to the boil, then simmer for 8–10 minutes, until reduced to a thin syrup. Stir in the cardamom and lemon juice.
6. Carefully spoon the syrup over the baked baklava, letting it seep into the walnut filling. Refrigerate until ready to serve.

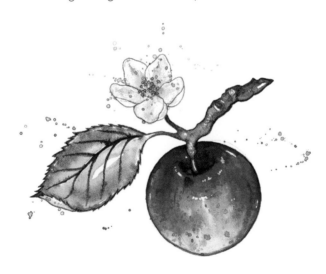

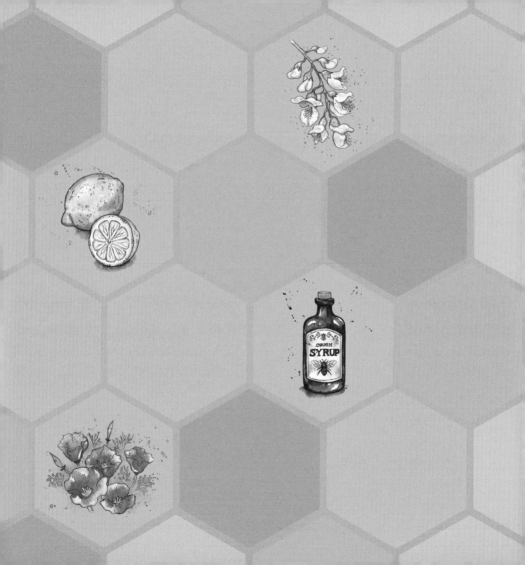

CHAPTER FIVE

HONEY HEALTHCARE AND BEAUTY RECIPES

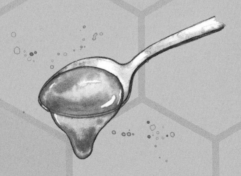

Honey is a miraculous multi-tasker when it comes to beauty treatments and healthcare. Both moisturizing and anti-bacterial, honey can be used by all skin types and ages to treat a variety of conditions or simply to maintain healthy skin. Despite its stickiness, it can also be used on hair to thicken and lighten it, as well as to heal the scalp and repair split ends.

Honey has been used to soothe sore throats and skin infections for millennia, but over the last decade it has enjoyed a real renaissance as the key ingredient in natural cough syrups for children. It is not recommended for infants under the age of one due to a bacteria potentially present in honey. Fortunately, this bacteria is harmless in the body after the age of one and does not interfere with the abundance of healing properties inherent in honey.

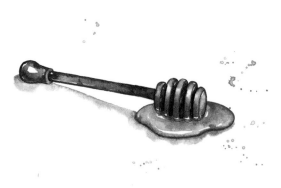

HONEY ON THE OUTSIDE

HAIR

Shampoo + Honey

The simplest way to benefit from the thickening, humectant qualities of honey without creating a sticky mess is to add it to your usual shampoo. Just as it feeds your body with vitamins and minerals, honey will also nourish your hair strands and scalp. Combine 1 tsp honey per penny-sized dollop of shampoo and lather as usual.

Multi-tasking Honey Cleanser

Serious honey aficionados and DIYers swear by their own honey shampoo created using nothing more than 1 tbsp honey and around 120ml (4fl oz) of warm water (double the recipe if needed). Shake them up in an empty bottle and you've got the world's sweetest hair wash! Since honey doesn't lather, squirt the mixture directly onto your scalp, massage gently, then rinse thoroughly. This concoction can also do double duty as an in-shower skin cleanser for both face and body.

Split Ends Repair

Honey mixed with olive or coconut oil (or any quality oil of choice) can be applied to split ends to increase softness and seal the hair cuticle. Simply combine ½ cup honey with ¼ cup olive oil or coconut oil. Apply it at night, keeping it under wraps and off your pillowcase with a shower cap, and rinse it out in the morning.

DIY Hair-lightening Treatment

Honey can lighten your hair and impart shine if you spray it with a mixture of 1 cup chamomile tea and 1 tbsp honey. Cover the hair with a shower cap and rinse it out in the morning. Continue the treatment weekly until the desired results are achieved.

Milk and Honey Hair Mask

Particularly beneficial for fine, brittle hair, a milk and honey mask imparts strength, volume, moisture and shine thanks to the keratin in honey and the protein, iron and zinc in milk. In a spray bottle, combine 250ml (8fl oz) skimmed milk with 1 tbsp honey. After shampooing, mist the hair with the spray bottle and let it soak into the hair for up to 20 minutes under a shower cap. Rinse out with warm water. There is no need to condition the hair.

Healthy Scalp Honey Treatment
Scalp conditions such as dandruff and dermatitis can benefit from a regular treatment of a honey and warm water mixture applied directly to the scalp from a spray bottle, separating the hair into sections as you would do when applying hair dye. Use a ratio of one part honey to two parts warm water, and allow the mixture to soothe the scalp for up to 20 minutes before rinsing.

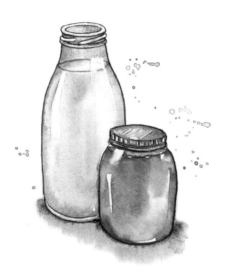

SKIN

Simple Honey Face Mask for All Skin Types
To treat dry, ageing skin, slather a tablespoon of honey over the entire face. Let it soak in for as long as is convenient, then rinse with warm water. To spot-treat acne flare-ups, apply a thin layer of honey over the affected area. For a deep, overnight treatment, particularly good for scars, cover with a bandage and rinse with warm water in the morning.

Honey Face Cream
This simple recipe has been used for thousands of years. Heat 110g (4oz) beeswax in a double boiler on low until melted. Stir in 250g (9oz) honey and 1 tbsp almond oil. Remove from the heat and stir until the mixture cools. Store in a jar with a tight-fitting lid.

Blackheads
A mixture of honey and lemon juice can be used as a blackhead treatment. For a single treatment, combine the juice of ½ lemon and 1 tsp honey. At night, apply to the affected area with a cotton ball as with an astringent.

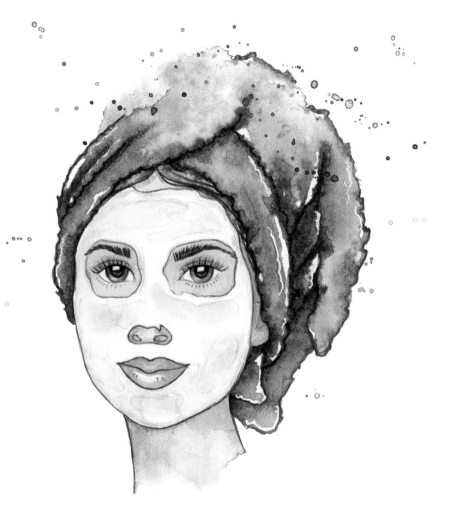

Honey Glow Facial Mask

Combine the tightening effects of aloe vera with the glowy and humectant effects of honey for a youth-imparting beauty mask. Mix one part honey with two parts pure aloe vera gel and apply any time of day or night, then rinse off after half an hour.

Honeyed Lips

Let honey soak into your lips overnight for a softer, sweeter pout in the morning by smoothing a thin layer of honey onto exfoliated lips at bedtime.

Wounds and Burns

Both animal and human wounds and burns can be treated with a dollop of honey to speed up healing. Thanks to its cell-regeneration powers, manuka or tea tree honey in particular is selected as an excellent natural topical treatment by dermatologists and veterinarians alike. It not only soothes the surface of the skin and relieves pain, but also shortens the healing process, helps prevent infection and reduces the chance of scarring. Gently apply raw honey to the affected area after cleaning and drying it, then cover with a bandage.

Findings from 2010 and 2019 trials documented in the NIH National Library of Medicine suggest honey dressings applied to diabetic foot ulcers effectively promoted healing quicker than conventional dressings. Further research is being conducted. The practice of using honey-impregnated dressings for healing wounds has been documented since 3000 BC. The preservation of bodies – mummification – by the Egyptians may have contributed to their knowledge of honey wrappings for wound treatment.

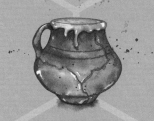

DID YOU KNOW?

Homeopaths and veterinarians often use manuka honey as an alternative natural treatment for use against infection. A medical-grade variation is used around the world for woundcare treatment; however, clinical trials have yet to prove its medical effectiveness.

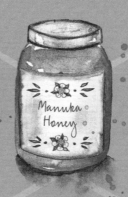

HONEY ON THE INSIDE

Ingesting honey is not only delicious, it actually improves your health! Rich in bioactive plant compounds and antioxidants that boost your immune system, it is easy to make a case for honey as a healthy substitute to sugar, which has zero health benefits and causes a variety of woes, including diabetes. While honey is a type of sugar, it is a natural sugar made from flower nectar and is more easily digested by the body. Though it still should be consumed in moderation by individuals who must watch their blood sugar levels, real raw honey is a safe treat for almost anyone, and a far better alternative to processed sweeteners.

Cough Syrup
The most common therapeutic use for honey across the millennia has been as welcome relief from a sore, scratchy throat. A few tablespoons in a cup of herbal tea or hot toddy (see pages 81 and 77) is a most pleasant way to soothe a cold or cough, without any of the side-effects of over-the-counter medicines. For a thicker syrup, stir honey slowly into roughly 120ml (4fl oz) of warm water until you reach your desired consistency. Swallow by the spoonful or sip in small doses.

COUGH MEDICINE

Pour 250ml (8fl oz) hot water over 1 tsp lemon juice, 1 tbsp honey and 3 cloves in a cup. Steep for 3 minutes then remove the cloves, stir and serve.

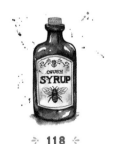

As a rule, the darker the honey, the more healing benefits it is believed to possess. The mix of organic acids and phenolic compounds gives honey its antioxidant punch. Studies have assessed the effectiveness of dark buckwheat honey in increasing antioxidant levels in the blood, reducing the risk of heart attacks and strokes. Reviews show that honey may play a promising role in reducing cardiovascular diseases, but there is no proven scientific evidence to date.

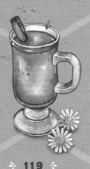

DID YOU KNOW?

Hippocrates, the fourth-century BC physician considered the founding father of Western medicine, wrote his own view of honey as a cure-all, writing, 'It cleans sores and ulcers, softens hard ulcers of the lips, heals carbuncles and running sores.'

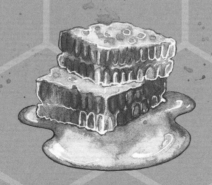

Energy Drink Alternative

Honey is a great natural alternative to all those energy-boosting concoctions so popular today. Honey is a sugar and carbohydrate like those energy drinks, but unlike those drinks it also contains fructose, which delivers energy more slowly than sucrose and without the crash after the high. Honey converts to a stored carbohydrate in the body, helping muscles maintain glycogen to draw upon when they need it. Just mix a spoonful of honey into a large glass of warm water, which will also help replenish your energy if you are fatigued due to dehydration.

Prebiotic

As opposed to antibiotics, which treat existing infections, or probiotics, which build up good bacteria to counter the bad, honey acts as a prebiotic, stimulating the growth of healthy bacteria in the gut. Adding raw honey to foods rich in probiotics, such as Greek yogurt, is like adding fertilizer to garden soil. Honey is a proven treatment against the *Helicobacter pylori* bacteria, a common cause of stomach ulcers.

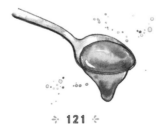

Allergy Relief

Eat local honey. You have probably heard of this folk remedy for seasonal allergies and it's worth a try: eat a large spoonful of raw honey every day, making sure that your honey was made from the pollen you are allergic to, and is from the area where you experience your symptoms. It's a natural way to build immunity to the allergen.

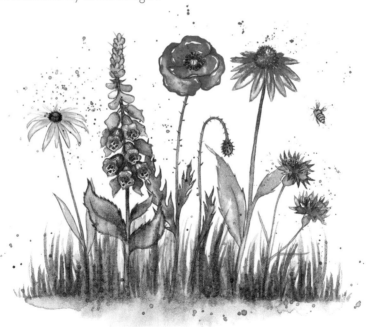

DID YOU KNOW?

Honey contains a variety of vitamins, minerals, amino acids and antioxidants in the form of flavonoids and phenolic acids. The floral source and its purity determines the amount and type of nutrients.

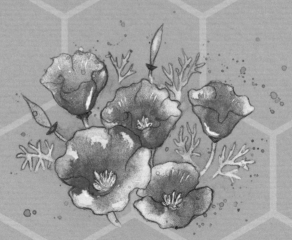

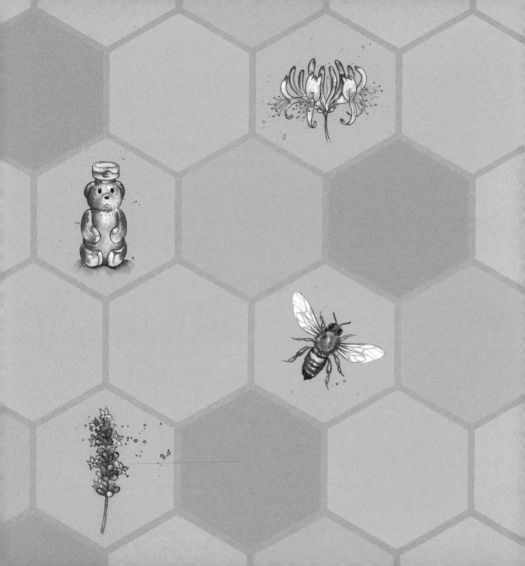

CHAPTER SIX

HONEY WISDOM

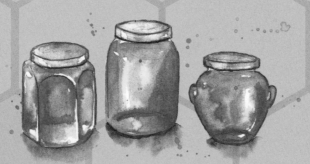

Now what delight can greater be
Than secrets for to knowe
Of Sacred Bees, the Muses' Birds,
All which this booke doth showe.

Charles Butler

Instead of dirt and poison, we have decided
to fill our hives with honey and wax; thus
furnishing mankind with the two noblest of
things, which are sweetness and light.

Jonathan Swift

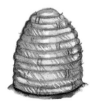

Honey comes out of the air ... At early dawn the leaves of trees are found bedewed with honey ... Whether this is the perspiration of the sky or a sort of saliva of the stars, or the moisture of the air purging itself, nevertheless it brings with it the great pleasure of its heavenly nature. It is always of the best quality when it is stored in the best flowers.

Pliny

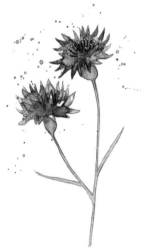

Tart words make no friends: a spoonful of honey
will catch more flies than a gallon of vinegar.

Benjamin Franklin

If you want to gather honey, don't
kick over the beehive.

Dale Carnegie

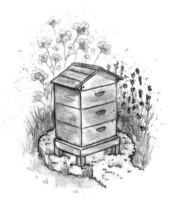

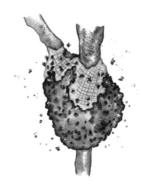

When you go in search of honey you must expect to be stung by bees.

Joseph Joubert

We are bees then; our honey is language.

Robert Bly

The honey is sweet, but the Bee stings.

George Herbert

Life is the flower for which love is the honey.

Victor Hugo

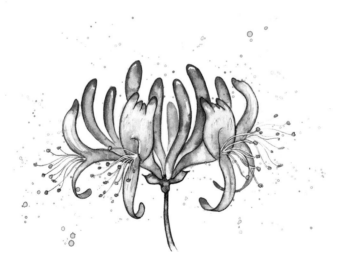

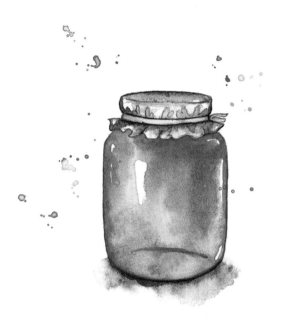

A day without a friend is like a pot without a single drop of honey left inside.

A. A. Milne (Winnie-the-Pooh)

We lived for honey. We swallowed a spoonful in the morning to wake us up and one at night to put us to sleep. We took it with every meal to calm the mind, give us stamina, and prevent fatal disease. We swabbed ourselves in it to disinfect cuts or heal chapped lips. It went in our baths, our skin cream, our raspberry tea and biscuits. Nothing was safe from honey . . . honey was the ambrosia of the gods and the shampoo of the goddesses.

Sue Monk Kidd, *The Secret Life of Bees*

The keeping of bees is like the direction of sunbeams.

Henry David Thoreau

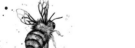

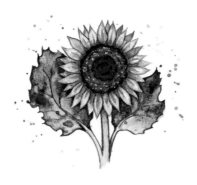

The bee collects honey from flowers in such a way as to do the least damage or destruction to them, and he leaves them whole, undamaged and fresh, just as he found them.

Saint Francis de Sales

A taste of honey is worse than none at all.

Smokey Robinson

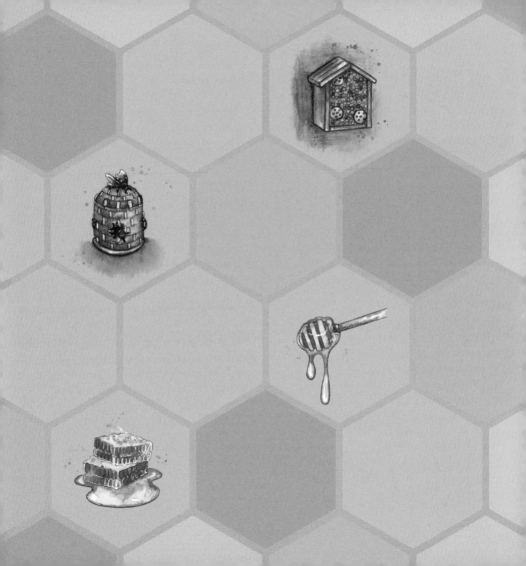

ADDITIONAL RESOURCES

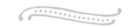

More Books on Honey and Bees

C. Marina Marchese and Kim Flottum, *The Honey Connoisseur: Selecting, Tasting and Pairing Honey*

Cal Orey, *The Healing Powers of Honey*

Charles Micucci, *The Life and Times of the Honeybee*

Colin G. Butler, *The World of the Honeybee*

Eva Crane, *A Book of Honey*

Hannah Nordhaus, *The Beekeeper's Lament: How One Man and Half a Billion Honey Bees Help Feed America*

HarperCollins, *Collins Beekeeper's Bible: Bees, honey, recipes and other home uses*

Hilary Kearney, *The Little Book of Bees: An Illustrated Guide to the Extraordinary Lives of Bees*

Holley Bishop, *Robbing the Bees: A Biography of Honey*

Jenni Fleetwood, *Honey: Nature's Magic – The Ultimate Practical Guide to 101 Things to Do with Honey, from Sweetening and Flavouring, to Polishing, Soothing and Healing*

Ron Fessenden, *The New Honey Revolution*

PODCASTS ABOUT HONEY

https://gastropod.com/the-buzz-on-honey/

https://www.keepingbackyardbees.com/harvest-your-honey-podcast-zepz2001ztil/

https://thehivejive.com/podcast/078-tasting-with-the-honey-sommelier/

https://www.norfolk-honey.co.uk/podcast/episode/49786177/episode-131-book-review-honey-by-dr-eva-crane

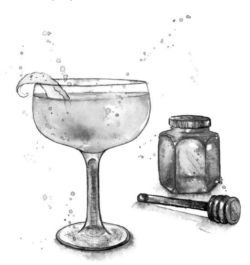

SELECT ONLINE RESOURCES TO LOCATE QUALITY HONEY, HONEY INFORMATION AND RECIPES

www.honeyassociation.com

www.bbka.org.uk/

www.americanhoneytastingsociety.com/

https://honey.com/

www.truesourcehoney.com

www.honeytraveler.com

https://apiarymap.com/

https://apiservices.pro

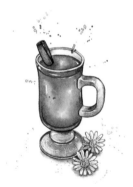

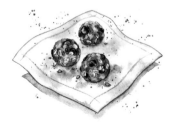

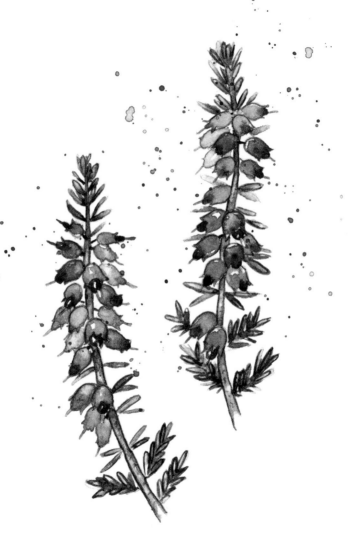

ACKNOWLEDGEMENTS

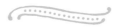

Thanks go to Caitlin Doyle for pitching this writing project on a topic dear to my heart. I am so fortunate to work with you! Thank you for your consistent professionalism, enthusiasm and encouragement. Thanks also go to Rachel Malig and Helena Caldon for polishing up the manuscript. Thanks to the artist, Amy Holliday, for making the book beautiful, and to Jacqui Caulton for the lovely design.

My husband, Tony Assaf, and his father, Kalim Assaf, are the brave beekeepers and cooks who introduced me to the fascinating and delicious world of beekeeping and honey. You are natural-born agrarians and providers; thank you for turning my romantic idea of the Milk and Honey Homestead into a reality.

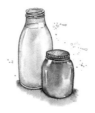

ABOUT THE AUTHOR

Andrea Kirk Assaf and her family keep dairy goats and honeybees on a farm in central Michigan that they have nicknamed The 'Milk and Honey Homestead', where life is frequently sticky and messy but always sweet. They were inspired to begin beekeeping by Kalim, the author's father-in-law, who first tended bees on the rooftop of his residence on Mount Lebanon. One day when Andrea's family was visiting, the colony split and the bees swarmed, clustering on a tree branch on a busy street. Incredibly, Kalim captured the swarm and moved the hives to a nearby monastery, where both the bees and the neighbours were more content.

The Homestead's bees have also provided a number of adventures, including curing a friend of apiphobia and treating allergies, as well as an organic wildflower honey business for a number of years. When many of the hives died one fateful winter, the business ended but the empty bee boxes were later colonized by wild bees, keeping the honey supply flowing and the farm pollinated. Andrea tries her best to practise what she preaches in this book, consuming honey first thing in the morning in her coffee and last thing in the evening in her tea, baking it into her bread, slathering it on her face, and mixing it in her shampoo. When not immersed in honey, Andrea home-schools her four children and writes books.

ABOUT THE ILLUSTRATOR

Amy Holliday is a freelance artist and illustrator based in Cumbria, England. In 2011, Amy graduated from the University of Cumbria with a BA (Hons) degree in illustration. Since then, she has worked on a wide variety of international projects, including children's and adult books, biological illustration, packaging from food to beauty, and much more. She works primarily in graphite and watercolours, before completing the piece digitally. She spends most of her days in her cosy home studio. When Amy is not working on a commission, she is creating her own work inspired by her latest fascination. Her favourite subjects to illustrate are all things related to the natural world. Other than art, Amy is passionate about wildlife conservation and environmentalism. She runs her own Etsy store, where she sells fine-art prints and products featuring her illustrations. You can find her online at www.amyholliday.co.uk.

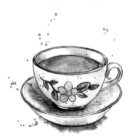

INDEX

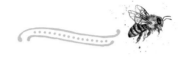

Page references in *italics* indicate images.

acacia honey 33
alfalfa honey 33
allergies 62, 122
amino acids 55, 123
antibiotics 48, 49, 53, 116, 121
antimicrobial properties 17, 45
antioxidants 55, 117, 119, 123
Apis mellifera (honey bee) 27
Apple Baklava Bites 104–105
apple blossom honey 33
artisan honey 30
aster honey 34
Avicenna 20
avocado honey 32, 34
Ayurvedic medicine 20

basswood honey 34
beer, honeyed 24
beechwood honey 34
beekeeper, befriending a 61–62
beeswax 11, 12, 112
bee worship 20, 21
blackberry honey 34
blackheads 112
blueberry honey 35
Bly, Robert 129
buckwheat honey 32, 35, 36, 119
Buddhist monks 23, 25
burial rituals 21, 25, 115
Butler, Charles 126

Café Miel 82, *83*
Carnegie, Dale 128
carrot honey 35
categories, honey 31
centrifugal honey extractor 10, *10*
chestnut honey 35
China 18, 25, 30, 35, 48, 49

Chinese tallow tree honey 35
Cleanser, Multi-tasking Honey 109
clover honey 36
coffee 80, 81
coffee blossom honey 36
comb honey 45
cough syrup 108, 118

dark buckwheat honey 119
Democritus 20
diabetic foot ulcers 115
Dionysus 20
DOP (*Denominazione di Origine Protetta*/ Protected Designation of Origin) label 30
drone bee *14*, 15

Egypt, ancient 18, 21, 22, 23, 24, 25, 115
energy drink alternative 121
etymology, honey 10
eucalyptus honey 32, 36

European Union 49, 61
Honey Directive 61

Face Cream, Honey 112
Face Mask for All Skin Types, Simple Honey 112
Facial Mask, Honey Glow 114
fermentation 17, 18
field bee 16, 17
filtered honey 32, 52
fireweed honey 36
flavonoids 123
flavours 28–45
foraging 16, 32, 36, 56
forms of honey, different 45
foulbrood disease 48
Franklin, Benjamin 128
Fruit Smoothie 71
FSA (UK Food Standards Agency) 49

Goat's Cheese, Honey and Fruit Crostini 84–85
gods, food of the 19–26
Gold Rush 72, *73*
goldenrod honey 36

hair 109–111
Hair-lightening Treatment, DIY 110
Hair Mask, Milk and Honey 110
Hapi, Nile god 23
harvesting 11

healthcare and beauty recipes 106–123
Healthy Scalp Honey Treatment 111
heather honey 43, 37
Helicobacter pylori bacteria 121
Herbert, George 130
Hippocrates 20, 120
Hittite Code 21
honey bee
 future of 26
 Latin name (*Apis mellifera*) 27
Honey-Brined Grilled Prawns 96–98
Honey Cake with Honey Buttercream Icing 102–103, *103*
honey cells 17
Honey-Garlic Pork Chops 94
Honey-Ginger Lemonade Punch 67
Honey Haddock 95
honey laundering 48, 49, 50
Honey-Lemon Dressing 89
Honey-Lime Chicken Skewers 91
honeymoon 18
honey production 12, 13
honey rituals 21
honey sac (crop) 16
Honey-Soy Salad Dressing 88
honey stomach (ventriculus) 16, 17
honey syrup 66

house bee 16, 17
Hruschka, Major Franz Elder von 10
Hugo, Victor 130
hydrogen peroxide 17, 45

immune system 117
International Honey Commission 61
invertase 17

Joubert, Joseph 129

land 'flowing with milk and honey' (Exodus 33:3) 23
lavender honey 37
lehua honey 37
linden honey 37
lips, honeyed 114
local honey 31, 32, 62, 122
London Honey Awards 61

macadamia honey 37
Madhu, festival of 23
manuka honey 39, 42, 114, 115, 116
marriage contracts 24
Maya's Honeyed Hot Cocoa *68*, 69–70
mead 18, 24, 37
melipona honey 39
melissopalynology (science of pollen analysis in honey) 58, 59

mellified man 25, 26
mesquite honey 40
microfiltration 52
Milne, A. A. 131
Monk Kidd, Sue: *The Secret Life of Bees* 132
multi-flower honey 31
mummification 21, 115
mythology and folklore 19, 20–27

National Honey Board 67, 77
nectar 16, 17, 30, 31, 32, 35, 36, 39, 42, 45, 48, 57, 61, 117
turning to honey 17
New Zealand 30, 34, 39
No-bake Honey Energy Bites 99–100, *101*

online resources 137
orange blossom honey 40
organic honey 56, 57, 119

palmetto honey 40
pasteurized honey 45, 54, 55
pesticides 32, 56
phenolic acids 123
Pliny 127
podcasts 136
pollen 11, 13, 16, 51, 53, 56, 59, 61, 62, 122
local 61–62

prebiotic 121
processing techniques 45
Prosciutto Honey Wraps 86–87
Pythagoras 20

queen bee *14*, 15

Ra (god of the created world) 21, 22
Ramses II, Pharaoh 23
raw (unheated) honey 10, 32, 45, 48, 51, 54, 55, 61, 114, 117, 121, 122
'real' honey 48–49
recipes
food and drink 64–105
healthcare and beauty 106–123

sage honey 32, 40
Sales, Saint Francis de 133
shades, honey 45
Shampoo + Honey 109
single-origin honey 31
skin 112–116
Smokey Robinson 133
sourwood honey 41
Spiced Hot Honey Toddy 77, *78*, 79
Split Ends Repair 110
Stout and Honey Beef Roast 92–93
Sumerian civilization 21

sunflower honey 41
superbugs 116
Swift, Jonathan 126

taxes 24
tea 36, 37, 80, 81, 118
The Bee's Knees 72, 74, 75–76
Thoreau, Henry David 132
thyme honey 41
Tony's Crazy Tea 81
true source certified 61
True Source Honey programme 61
tupelo honey 32, 42

ulmo honey 42
ultrafiltration 51–52, 53
ultraviolet vision 16
United States 30, 34, 35, 36, 40, 41
unpasteurized honey 54, 55, 61

Versatile Honey-Mustard Sauce 90
vitamins 123

whipped honey 45
wildflower, or polyfloral, honey 31, 32, 42
worker bee 13, *14*, 15, 16
wounds and burns 114

Zeus 20